To Run The Race
With Joy

*Since we are surrounded by
such a great cloud of witnesses,
let us ... run with perseverance
the race marked out for us.*
Hebrews 12:1

Sandy Rice

CSS Publishing Company, Inc., Lima, Ohio

TO RUN THE RACE WITH JOY

Library of Congress Cataloging-in-Publication Data

Rice, Sandy, 1943-
    To run the race with Joy / by Sandy Rice.
        p.   cm.
    ISBN 0-7880-1064-6
    1. Breast—Cancer—Patients—Religious life. 2. Seales, Joy—Religion. 3. Breast—Cancer—Patients—Biography. 4. Seales, Joy—Health. I. Title.
BV4910.33.R53   1997
248.8'6196994—dc21   96-51817
                                                                                    CIP

ISBN: 0-7880-1064-6   PRINTED IN U.S.A.

DEDICATION

I dedicate this book to my loving husband, Jim. His encouragement, support, and unselfish love through this time in our lives has been a most cherished gift from God. His love is a perfect example of 1 Corinthians 13, and I will never cease to thank God for him. He is God's greatest treasure to me!

In Appreciation

First, I want to thank my husband Jim, and our children, Andrew, Adam, Julie and Rita, for their love and understanding during these past five years. Special thanks to Jim and Andrew for their patience with a computer illiterate wife and mother. I couldn't have completed this work, at least not in this century, without their help. And last, but not least, I thank my dear mother who first taught me the love of Jesus Christ!

I want to thank our friends and members of Grace Brethren Church, Alexandria, Virginia and Faith Evangelical Presbyterian Church of Kingstowne, Virginia. Without your encouragement and prayer support we could not have survived.

I am especially grateful to Debbie Smith and Debbie Weidman for their love and for the many hours they have so graciously given in the promotion of this book.

To Dr. Katherine Alley and Dr. Roy Beveridge: God blessed you with marvelous skills and compassionate hearts. I am so thankful that He placed you in Joy's life.

To our friends and co-workers at NBC Studios in Washington, D.C., Thomas A. Edison High School in Alexandria, Virginia, and the Fairfax County Health Department, who have been so supportive to Joy and to me during these past years.

And finally, to CSS Publishing for giving me the wonderful opportunity to share this story.

Introduction

This is a unique story of a friendship, through tragedy and triumph.
It's a story of laughter, tears and pain.
It's a story of family, hope and love.
It's a story of sacrifice, perseverance and faith.
It's a story of victory.
It's a story of Joy.

Preface
By
Joy Seale

Living with cancer has changed my life in many ways. The most important change has been a deeper relationship to the Lord Jesus Christ. I have learned to depend on Him and to desire, above all, to be more like Him. Cancer is not my life. It is just a diversion from the real purpose of my life which is to glorify Jesus Christ! But if I can best accomplish this through my cancer, then I accept that — to God be the glory!

I want to thank my mother for teaching me through her own battle with cancer how to fight and never give up ... even to the end. Mom, I miss you and without your faith and strength as an example, I would not be the person I am today. Thank you for being my mother! I love you!

How do I thank my best friend, Sandy, for sticking by me through the toughest challenge of my life? I have always been a person who prides herself in being able to handle anything and everything that life has to offer, but cancer isn't something that I could face alone! I was never able to share my illness with my mother because I realized that seeing me with cancer broke her heart, for she knew firsthand what the future might hold for me. Therefore, I relied on my friend, Sandy, for support and companionship during this time of my life. She is a friend who could only have been given to me by God. There are many types of friends but she became more than a friend. She became my "family" and she got involved. Not because she had to, it was her choice! I thank God for her willingness, and her family's willingness, to become a part of my life. Sandy has always been there when I needed her, asking no questions!

7

When God is the central part of a friendship, the friendship is taken into another dimension that the world does not understand. God has blessed our friendship and has caused it to grow through my illness. Thank you, Lord, for allowing me to have one of your most precious blessings from above — my friend, Sandy!

To Sandy: If I had only one friend left, I'd want it to be you!

Love, Joy!

Comments

JOY SEALE is one of the most courageous, brave, and enthusiastic people I know. She is full of life and love and laughter — and that makes all the difference — not only to herself but to all those around her. She is a warrior with great compassion and great faith who is willing to share the experiences of her continuing battle with cancer to help others understand theirs.

Willard Scott
NBC News

Joy Seale is a woman of incredible strength, courage, and optimism. Her story is awe inspiring. It tells of Joy's unshakable faith and the power of an extraordinary friendship.

Katie Couric
NBC News

If I were to read this fascinating story without knowing the real-life people involved, I might be tempted to think that the author has exaggerated (unconsciously, of course) by adding a note of triumph to every trial and a humorous sparkle to suffering. The story has an innocent, childlike beauty that we want to believe ... but can't because we live in a real world where skepticism is the rule.

The truth is that I know Joy Seale, her friend Sandy Rice and Sandy's enthusiastic, supportive family, and I must say in the words of the Queen of Sheba, "The half has not been told."

Sandy believes that the grace of God is the only real thing in this world, and that trusting Him provides an experience worth reporting. This is the story of how God is delighting to work in the lives of two of His delightful children.

Dean I. Walter
Retired Chemist and Elder
Grace Brethren Church
Clinton, Maryland

Joy could not have been more appropriately named. I have considered it a privilege to be involved in her care. Here is a woman battling breast cancer with the ability to make people laugh. She actually had me *laughing on the way to the operating room. I do not think you can be involved with her and not develop a sense of real attachment. One of her first questions after surgery was, when could she play softball! Such courage and love of living should serve as an inspiration to us all.*

Katherine Alley, M.D., F.A.C.S.

10

*It has been said that "Imitation is the sincerest form of flattery."
If that is true then I would covet the lessons learned (but without
having to go through the process) by both Joy Seale and Sandy
Rice. While wholeheartedly submitting to God's greater glory in
their lives, both disciple and mentor have gained invaluable
insights. First, that God in his creation has allowed the mantle of
suffering to be set upon certain of His choice servants. Those
ministers of/in suffering uniquely demonstrate the qualities of His
grace. Both Joy and Sandy have borne well this mantle and will
touch the life of the reader as a result. Second, suffering is an
exacting teacher and a demanding communicator. The admission
to the course taught is costly, but the benefits are great. It was said
of Christ that "he offered up prayers and petitions with loud cries
and tears to the one who could save him from death, and he was
heard because of his reverent submission ... he learned obedience
from what he suffered...." As a pastor and friend, I commend both
Joy and Sandy for their lessons learned and shared with the same
openness and transparency that Oliver Cromwell once declared
upon viewing his portrait, "Do it over, warts and all."*

Robert A. Trefry, Former Pastor-Teacher
Grace Brethren Church
Alexandria, Virginia

*Having treated and cared for Joy these many years, I agree
completely with the thoughts in this book of:*

*Being active — Joy with her boundless energy,
Purpose — Cancer does not rule Joy's life, and
Friendship — With her family, adopted family, and those she comes
in contact with.*

Roy A. Beveridge, M.D.

I cannot enthusiastically enough commend Sandy Rice for the manner in which, in this inspirational narrative, she has portrayed the radiant, triumphant faith and indomitable courage of a young Christian woman, Joy Seale, a devoted member of our congregation here in Alexandria, Virginia, who continues to wage unrelenting warfare against a stubborn disease.

The Bible never attempts to explain *suffering, but it does give us example after example of how suffering can be* faced, accepted, *and* conquered *in the power of the risen Christ.*

We reflect upon what the Apostle Paul wrote in 2 Corinthians 12:7-9: "To keep me from becoming conceited ... there was given me a thorn in my flesh*" (Paul doesn't tell us what it was, so that every sufferer might be able to relate to his dilemma), "a messenger of Satan, to torment me. Three times I pleaded with the Lord to take it away from me. But He said to me, 'My* grace is sufficient for you, for My power is made perfect in weakness.' Therefore I will boast all the more gladly about my weaknesses, so that Christ's power may rest on me.... *"*

Those of us who are privileged to know Joy Seale can assure you that she is indeed a living testimony not only to the saving and life-transforming power of Christ, but also that the Lord has done for Joy what He has done for that countless number of believers who have had to face adversity, often in its direct forms — He has given her the inner resources of the Spirit to be what Paul calls "more than conquerors" *(Romans 8:37). She knows that Jesus never promises to make life* easy *for those who follow Him; but He does promise to make us* strong *to face life courageously and triumphantly, and in Joy's case, almost cavalierly.*

Your hearts will be blessed and your faith enriched as you meet Joy in the pages of this splendid and challenging book. The Christian world is deeply indebted to Mrs. Rice for the vivid portrait she has painted of an outstanding young contemporary Christian who, in spite of justifiable doubts and fears, continues to "do justly, love mercy, and walk humbly with her God" (Micah 6:8).

William Graham Smith, Pastor Emeritus
Faith Evangelical Presbyterian Church
Alexandria, Virginia

Joy Seale has faced breast cancer with grace and dignity and humor. By doing that, she has given those of us who are lucky enough to work with her at NBC News a chance to learn how to face adversity with less fear and more faith. It is a privilege to be her friend.

Terry Schaefer
Today Show Producer
NBC News

This wonderful book about Joy's struggle is a daily reminder of God's goodness, and the power of prayer. Watching over and working with Joy has taught me how to accept life's challenges without being overcome or defeated. She is my friend, my child and my Joy.

Phyllis J. Law, Supervisor
Electronic Journalism
NBC, Washington, D.C.

I am a Social Worker who helps patients and families cope with the devastating effects of life-threatening illness ... The truth is cancer often leaves patients asking "who am I now?" and caregivers feeling helpless and trapped. Life-threatening illness pushes people to their limit mentally, physically, emotionally, and spiritually. There are often more questions left than answers.

However, Joy's story is a testimony of hope — it is a battle that is won by how she chooses to live. It gives people a choice at a time when most choices have been taken away, and it teaches all of us what living is truly about.

Joy's story is about what cancer can't do, and about what God can.

Nicole J. Armes, M.S.S.W.

13

As a registered nurse, I have firsthand knowledge in dealing with illness and the people it involves. Caregivers have an extremely difficult role as they must deal with multiple issues. They care for the person who is ill while continuing to care for their own families and homes. Most caregivers also work outside their homes. Caregivers make sure the patients get to doctors' appointments, they learn to give treatments at home, they see the patients through surgeries, hospitalization and all the while trying to get their own needs met. For a caregiver who is not a family member, the role is even more difficult.

Sandy Rice became that kind of caregiver. Without the support of her husband, her children and mother, I don't think Sandy could have done all that she did for her friend. To meet her own needs, Sandy wrote a story; to meet the needs of others, she wrote a book. To Run The Race With Joy *will touch the hearts of many, whether in the role of caregiver, family or friend. It is not about sadness; it's a story about friendship, family, love, faith, disappointments and Joy.*

Harriet Zimmerman, R.N., B.S.N.
Public Health Nurse
Fairfax County Health Department
Fairfax, Virginia

As a Christian, this book has really touched my heart in a very special way, and has served to bring my family closer together, even though we have not gone through this type of crisis. I believe it has taught me how to become more of a servant to my family. I want to encourage others to read this inspiring story so that their families may also be strengthened in Christ. It is a blessing to work with Sandy, my sister in the Lord, and to know her family and through her to know her friend, Joy.

Pamela Keith
Thomas A. Edison High School
Alexandria, Virginia

Chapter 1

The Diagnosis

Exhausted from yet another trip to the doctor to find out why my legs ache all the time, I turned on my answering machine. "Yesss!" a flippant voice cried out. "I can go to the beach for the entire week! I know you were secretly hoping for a few days without me," she said sarcastically, "but ha, ha, I fooled you! Well, bye. Talk to you later. Love ya." She had so hoped she could go to the beach with our family as she had done for the past six years. However, due to her schedule of radiation therapy, she didn't know until today, only two days before we were to leave, that she indeed could go with us. I prayed and thanked God for yet another wonderfully answered prayer on my friend's behalf. My own aches and pains were quickly put back into perspective, and I began to thank Him for my nagging bursitis!

"Cancer." The word is so frightening! However, Joy and I had learned a lot about it in the last two years — more than we had ever intended.

It was on her thirty-fifth birthday in July of 1991, that she decided she could no longer ignore the lump in her right breast. I had been urging her to go to the doctor for weeks, but she felt that the lump could have been caused by an injury she had suffered at work some weeks before, and she just kept hoping it would go away by itself. You see, Joy is very stubborn, and extremely hard-headed! However, I, too, can be equally stubborn, so she soon tired of my constant hassle, relented, and made an appointment to see a doctor.

Neither one of us, ever in a hundred years, expected this to be anything except something simple. We joked and had our usual off-the-wall humorous conversation while we waited in the doctor's office to get the results of her mammogram. Consequently, we were totally unprepared when the doctor told her the lump was a tumor, most assuredly malignant, and immediate surgery was definitely required! I can't explain our reaction except to say that even though we were in total shock, we still, I believe, were also in complete denial, because we just couldn't believe that this could actually be breast cancer — not the breast cancer that is really, really serious! I mean not that all breast cancer isn't serious, but other women have been cured and have beaten it, so there was no reason to doubt that Joy could not have the same end result, if it indeed was truly breast cancer! We never really considered any possibility other than, number one, it was a mistake, or number two, it would turn out to be something very simple and very easy to fix!

We reasoned that we could do this! We would get the best surgeon (if a second opinion confirmed the first one), there would be lots of prayer, which we never doubted, she would only have to have a lumpectomy, not a mastectomy, there would be no cancerous lymph nodes involved (the doctor had told her this was a possibility), and it would be, as we thought it would be, a simple thing, easily resolved! Right?

We turned it over to the Lord there and then. We would get through this together with Him, and it would be all right again, very soon! Little did we know that this was only to be the first battle in her war with "serious" breast cancer!

Giving her mother the test results was very difficult, because she herself had been living with cancer, lymphoma, for over fourteen years. Joy had been living at home with her mother since her graduation from college. As much as she had wanted to move out into a place of her own, she just couldn't bring herself to do it, because she couldn't fathom the thought of her mother living alone with cancer. Due to circumstances in her family, Joy had pretty much become the "mother" for most of her life, and it was a role that she had come to accept. She had put her own desires on "hold," and trusted God to help her to cope with the problems that came with that situation. And indeed, she had handled it very well.

Her mother took the news as well as could be expected. A few days later, as we waited together during Joy's breast surgery, we talked and prayed together. The love for her child was evident by the pain on her face. Your child is supposed to outlive you, as a parent, and the possibility of facing the worst scenario did not seem normal. How could she cope with her own cancer, let alone that of her child? Opal had, only in the last few years, come back into fellowship with the Lord, so I knew she needed extra special prayer, lest she stumble. "God," I prayed, "give strength to all of us at this very moment. We need your presence as never before. Opal needs your encouragement and shelter from this impending storm. Cover her now with your everlasting arms, and let her feel you close to her." I knew my husband, my family, and our church were even at this moment praying for all of us. The wait seemed like an eternity, but I felt their prayers and God's presence as we waited....

Chapter 2

In The Beginning

Next to my husband Jim, Joy is my best friend, even with our thirteen-year age difference. Jim and I were youth leaders in our church for several years, and I had the privilege of leading her to the Lord when she was fourteen years old. For the next two years after that, I discipled her, and our family and church loved her as we saw her begin to grow in the Lord. Having come from a non-traditional family, Joy thrived on all the love the people showed to her. She had even expressed a desire to perhaps become a missionary. However, when she was sixteen years old, due to problems in her family, she left our church. All contact with our family or the church family was cut off. We all prayed for her, knowing that she needed much guidance and discipline in order to keep her life focused in the right direction. It became increasingly difficult to keep in contact because of family pressure. I did continue to write letters for awhile, until it became abundantly clear that I could no longer do that. I just had to rely on prayer.

Then one Sunday, after having not seen her or having no contact with her in almost seven years, I looked up to see her walk into our church again! She looked like the little lost girl we had first seen when she was only fourteen. She had graduated from college in Tennessee, had a job at NBC studios in Washington, D.C., and still lived in the area with her family. Now, as an adult, she was free to choose for herself her friends and her church, and she was exercising that freedom.

Unfortunately, it was just as I had feared. She told me she had strayed far from the Lord during those years, even though she had attended a Christian college. She confessed she had been involved in much sin and had acquired some less-than-desirable habits. When I told her we had been praying for her all along, she said she believed that must have been the reason she had been kept from even more evil in her life, for she had not fallen, by the grace of God, into sex or drugs. She tearfully thanked me for praying and for our unconditional love, and expressed her desire to have me disciple her once again ... she wanted to make a new commitment to Christ!

It was a long and sometimes painful process, but the Lord always forgives and never gives up on us; so as the months and years went by, we began to see her mature in Him and become His witness.

Over those years, she grew from a student to a friend and, because of her love for the Lord and our family and because of her own family situation, we sort of "adopted" her. Our boys, Andrew and Adam, adore her, and she dotes on them like a sister. She never actually "grew up," which of course pleases them. She is always the life of the party, full of fun and good-natured mischief. She is sometimes exasperating, sometimes unpolished, sometimes hot-tempered, and sometimes, ever so briefly, slips a bit back into her old ways. Of course, I am usually there to chastise her and she still to this day tolerates my lectures very well.

Above all, Joy is the most unselfish and giving person I know. She loves the Lord fiercely, and wants very much to please Him, so we continue to have "discipling" sessions from time to time. At other times, she winds up teaching me. Her battle with this disease has caused her to grow, in some ways well beyond her years.

Even from the beginning, she has never asked, "Why, Lord?" When she was first diagnosed with the cancer, I remember what she said: "Why not me? What makes me so special? I'd much rather it be me than you. You have Jim, the boys, and your mother. They need you. I will just trust the Lord. It will be all right. Don't worry." All who know her marvel at her strength and faith in the Lord. She has never blamed God! Never! Oh, we have certainly cried together many times ... cried because she never found the right guy, cried because she will never bear children, cried because she lost her hair, cried because she is too young to have this disease, but never has she cried because she doubted God or because she thought He was unfair. Not once! Through it all she has become more dependent on Him, more trusting, much more faithful, and, as a result, has been an inspiration to both Christians and non-Christians.

We have daily devotional books alike; however, more often than not, it is she who never skips a day. She has often chided me for forgetting to have my devotions, as she excitedly relates a passage from the day's devotional only to have me admit that I hadn't taken time to read it. "Oh, no," she would say, sounding so disappointed. "It fit the day so perfectly and it meant so much to me. Read it when you get home." Sure enough, I would read it only to find out that it would have gotten me through the day so much easier if I had taken the time to read it before the day had begun! I am made to realize that God is so faithful if we only allow Him to be. How can I neglect the reading of God's Word even though I see it giving her extraordinary strength?

I often have felt that her illness is unfair, and have at times questioned God, if only for a moment. My husband then reminds me of the fact that God has a plan, and as much as I like to "fix" everything for everyone (my family calls me "Miss Organizer," "Miss Social Director," or "Miss Fix-it"), I cannot "fix" this, and I must learn to let God have control and trust Him. I know I need His Word every day to give me wisdom and strength, but I still find I'm trying to rely on myself, and of course I fail, and then become totally frustrated. Why, I continually question myself, is giving Him control so hard to do, when I know it is the only thing that works? Why had I not learned to "trust in the Lord with all your heart and lean not on your own understanding; ... and He will make your paths straight" (Proverbs 3:5, 6)?

Chapter 3

Our Dad

My husband, Jim: how could I ever ask for a more perfect mate? He has been a rock. I know it's been hard sharing a wife with a friend who has required so much time and attention; but through it all he has been extremely supportive and understanding. He just takes all three of us, my mother who lives with us, Joy, and me, to our mountain retreat for a weekend, to dinner, or to the movies. You see, not only has he had to share my time with Joy, but with my mother as well. For the past twenty-one years, because of health problems, my mother, through Jim's invitation, has made her home with us. He has treated her like his own mother who died twenty-two years ago, and she, in turn, thinks of him as her own son. Cancer touched my mother in 1981, but early detection and surgery provided her a cure, and we are so grateful to God for sparing her life. She is a vital part of our family and has been such a positive influence on our children over the years. With the boys, their "Nina" is, and always will be, "Number 1."

Our "extended family" has worked beautifully through the years, and I thank God for the "give and take" that He has helped each one of us to develop in order to make it work. But I am especially thankful for Jim who seems to do most of the "giving" for all of us. It seems when he married me he got more than he bargained for, but we love each other more today than we did thirty-three years ago, and we have a marriage as perfect as you can get this side of heaven. His marvelous sense of humor, his tremendous wisdom, and most especially his relationship with the Lord have made our family what it is!

At times it seems unfair, but we all depend heavily on Jim, for he just seems to know the right thing to do. Maybe it's because he is an attorney and he is used to trying to negotiate and work things out for people, but he tries to put everything into the right perspective, and just seems to always have the right answer. In our family it's "Dad" who can do it all. It must put tremendous stress on him, and at times I can sense that it does, but he is always there for all of us, and I know deep inside he wouldn't have it any other way.

Joy considers Jim her "father," maybe because her relationship with her own father was nonexistent. Her father is the one area of her life that she is reluctant to discuss, even with me. Something happened in her childhood that evidently was very traumatic. Except for one brief conversation we had on the subject, I have never been able to get her to open up to me. I just prayed and knew that God alone would have to work it out for her. Sometimes we have to know when to back off and let God handle it. It is hard for me, "Miss Fix-it," to do that, but I'm trying.

Joy sends Father's Day cards to Jim and asks his advice on everything from her car to legal matters, as well as his opinion on politics and theology, for she, too, values his opinions, takes his advice, and loves him dearly. He has been utterly exasperated with her spending habits and her indulgence with our sons and our daughter-in-law, but of course, much as she values his opinion, she does have a strong will, and she simply says, "You are my second family and I can never repay you for what you have meant to me. This is my choice. End of conversation!" Of course this is said with that ever-present smile and twinkle in her eye, and you just know you will not win because she always has to have the last word!

Chapter 4

The War Begins

The doctor is here now — the long wait is over! She gives her mom and me the news. It is BREAST CANCER, with seven out of the fourteen lymph nodes tested being cancer-positive. The war had begun! We would be living with cancer — all of us! All of us who love and care for her will live with it. Those few "friends" and yes, even some relatives, who can't handle it, and abandon her, were never really friends at all.

I can't possibly construe my feelings! I felt myself going completely numb. My body tingled with a cold sense of fear, and yet I felt intensely hot! My throat felt like it was closing, and I couldn't speak because my mouth was suddenly painfully dry. I knew that I couldn't let go of my emotions just then, because Joy's mother needed me to be strong. It was only the Lord that enabled me to put them aside in order to take charge of the situation. God allowed me to be strong for Joy's mother when I felt inexplicably weak. His strength is perfect when our strength is gone, and never before had I felt this to be more true!

We listened as the doctor explained that she had performed a lumpectomy on Joy's right breast, and that despite the lymph node involvement, she had been able to obtain what is called "clear margins" around the mass. That meant she had removed the cancerous mass as well as areas surrounding the mass, therefore creating a clear margin all around the diseased area. That, she stated, was very important. She sounded optimistic. She is an excellent surgeon, highly respected in her field, and we were confident that she had done exactly the right procedure. She explained that Joy would need extensive chemotherapy, and she was making arrangements with top oncologists to see her when she was out of the hospital.

The word "chemotherapy" was very familiar to Opal because she had taken it for years. She sobbed uncontrollably at the prospect of her daughter having to go through the same thing. It was one of the hardest situations that I had ever faced. How could I comfort her? What could I possibly say that would ease her pain? We cried together, and then I simply reminded her that although I could not possibly understand, God did. He had watched his only Son suffer many times beyond anything we could ever imagine, even to death, and He would comfort her as nobody else could. She seemed to grasp and hold onto that thought as I prayed for us as well as for her child, my dearest friend!

We waited for Joy to be taken from the recovery room to her room, and then we were told we could go see her. "Lord," I prayed, "please give my friend the grace as never before to face this, her most difficult challenge. Keep Opal and me strong for her and give us wisdom."

I could not believe it when we walked into her room! She was her usual funny and upbeat self. "Things are going to be fine," she said, as we bent down to kiss her obviously tear-stained cheek. She had already been given the grace that we had sought for her. God was already at work in her spirit, and was preparing her for what would lie ahead. I thanked Him, realizing what a mighty God we do serve! Through Him, she had managed to comfort us instead of us comforting her! The Lord was her Comforter, and that was all she needed just then. He is sufficient!

Chapter 5

Curse Of The Cure

Chemotherapy! It is a word Joy hated because she had seen her mother suffer from its side effects for years. And yet it was the substance that had kept her mother alive for so long that it had amazed even the doctors. Each time she was told by her doctors that her time might be very short, a new type of chemotherapy would be tried, it would work, and she would go into remission again. Her mother was a fighter, and her "never give up" attitude had inspired Joy. As afraid as she was of the treatment, her response was, "My mother did it and survived, and so will I." We prayed about it, and she trusted the Lord to give her the same strength He had given to her mother.

The day arrived for her first treatment, and we went to the oncologist's office together. What a revelation! Cancer is no respecter of persons. Old, young, very young, men, women, children — they were all there. Women who had obviously lost their hair as a result of the treatment were there in their wigs and turbans. Husbands were there with their wives and wives with their husbands, giving much needed support. It was just a place we never thought we would be, and from the look on Joy's face as she glanced around the room, I knew she was terrified! I prayed and asked the Lord to give her peace and a calm assurance. I tried to joke with her as we sat down together after she had registered with the nurse. As hard as she tried to otherwise occupy her mind with anything except what she was about to face, it was apparent that she could not. Thankfully, it was not too long before a very pleasant nurse called her name and took us back to the treatment room.

I immediately realized this woman was just the kind of nurse Joy needed. She would be administering the chemotherapy for each of Joy's treatments. Her name, appropriately, was Sunny! Sunny was humorous, upbeat, obviously very good at her job, and took an instant liking to Joy. I thanked God because Joy seemed to be relaxing a bit, and her face seemed to reflect it. Sunny explained in great depth what she would be doing, and that each procedure would take about an hour to complete. I sat down beside the bed-chair and watched as she placed the first IV tube in Joy's arm.

"This first medication will take about twenty minutes," Sunny explained. "It is an anti-nausea medication called Zofran, that hopefully will keep you from getting sick after the chemo. It seems to work very well, and I have no doubt at all that it will work for you too. You will learn to love it." She made a funny face and laughed as she left the room. Once alone, Joy could no longer hold in the tears that up until that moment had been hidden.

"What will all this stuff do to the rest of my body?" she said, as the tears welled up in her eyes. "I feel so strange and so helpless! I've never before felt so helpless." "Miss Independent" had suddenly become very dependent, and that sense of losing control could clearly be seen by the look of fear in her eyes. I held her hand and prayed out loud for her, and asked God for His strength for her as well as for me. I just could not lose control at that time. She needed me to be strong for her.

"Oh, God," I prayed silently. "Give me your strength. I can't do it on my own." God's grace and strength were immediate! The nurse returned to finish the treatment, and by the time the hour was gone, with Joy's tremendous sense of humor and my ad libs, we had the nurses in stitches. They said they looked forward to our next visit, and while we couldn't exactly say we "looked forward" to seeing them again under these circumstances, I knew we would get through these treatments because God had answered prayer in a way that only He knew was best. I thanked Him for those nurses and their caring, positive attitude. I knew we could do this. I just knew it! And the best thing was that Joy knew it too!

"Do you want to participate in a study of a new drug that is being tested that will perhaps keep your white blood count up during your chemotherapy?" The question was posed to Joy by another nurse, Kathy, just as we were getting our calendar set up for Joy's subsequent treatments before leaving the doctor's office that first time. "If you choose to participate," she continued, "the injections will be free but, of course, we won't know whether you have been given a placebo or the real medication until after your treatments are completed. Even we don't know which patients are receiving the placebo, and which are receiving the real stuff. We have to wait just like you do." She had told us that this aggressive chemotherapy Joy was receiving would cause her white blood count to drop. The white blood cells are infection-fighting cells; therefore, if her white blood count were to drop too low, it could become dangerous for her, and she would possibly have to be hospitalized and given blood transfusions. In fact, Kathy explained, it was not only a possibility but a probability that hospitalization would be necessary at least once during her treatments. Knowing the facts, it didn't take long for Joy to agree to take part in the study. She was all in favor of anything that would keep her from having to go to the hospital. Kathy explained that the injections were to be given one a day, for ten days, on the third day following the chemotherapy, beginning with this first treatment she had just completed.

"Great!" Joy replied. "Do I come back here to get the shots?" Then the "kicker" was thrown in!

"No need for that! The injections are self-administered. I'll show you a video that will explain everything to you," Kathy said, sounding very confident that this would work.

"What?" Joy yelled, as she looked at me with that "she's got to be kidding" look. "I can't give myself a shot. No way! I just can't do it."

"Well, that's all right. Maybe someone in your family could do it for you," Kathy said, patting Joy's hand to calm her down. Joy and I both knew that was not a possibility at all. Her mother would be too nervous to do it, and no one else could. She turned and looked at me, and I instantly knew what she was thinking!

"Me?" I gasped. "Well, I guess I could learn to do it. It would, in fact, give me great pleasure to do it," I said jokingly. We all laughed, but inside I was virtually trembling! What if I couldn't do it? I had never before given an injection. I was trained to give injections to students who had bee sting allergies, but I had never actually had to inject anyone! I work at a high school as a health aide — Band-Aids, ice, TLC. I am not a nurse! I don't do shots! I realized that there simply was not anyone else. I had to do it, and I had to be confident and reassuring. So, I watched the video, asked lots of questions, practiced on an orange, and after convincing myself and the nurse that I could do it, we were given the ten syringes and the medication (placebo or real?), and we left. What, I quietly asked myself, had I gotten myself into? Oh well, I told God that He would have to handle this one too! And I knew He would!

Every day for ten days, on the third day following her chemotherapy treatment, she would stop at my house on her way home from work (yes, she went back to work as soon as the doctor would allow) and I would give her an injection. The first injection I gave was, of course, the scariest. My hand shook as I assured her that I remembered everything I had learned. Of course, I wasn't even sure I had learned anything, because it had only been three days since I had agreed to this crazy thing, and I was still in shock!

With the grace of God, we got through that first one, and then I actually got pretty good at it. Sometimes the injection itself hurt her, and sometimes it didn't. We could never figure it out. I only know that later on when she received the very same type of injections from registered nurses, Joy said the reaction was the same. Sometimes they hurt, and sometimes they didn't! At least I knew it wasn't me! After I had given forty injections, you would think it would have gotten easier, but it never did. I would sweat and swallow hard every time I had to do it. I hated each one of them, but knowing it was a way to help, a tangible and real way to help, made it much easier, and I considered it a privilege.

Chapter 6

Reality Sets In

I believe the worst part of these treatments was not the nausea, the diarrhea, the cramps, the feeling of weakness, or even the injections. It was losing her hair! Joy has beautiful, thick hair, and losing it was very difficult for her. When she started discovering loose hair in the shower, and handfuls of hair in her brush, she knew it was only a matter of time until she would lose it all. She was crying the day she called to tell me of the gobs of hair that were falling from her head! She then began experiencing headaches, as more and more hair began to come out. The weight of the now dead hair follicles on her head caused headaches.

One evening, she begged me, "Please just pull out all the hair from my head. I know it is all going to come out anyway, and I just want it over with so maybe I won't have the headaches." I couldn't believe what she was asking me to do for her, but on the other hand, I also couldn't stand the look of desperation on her face. So, as she sat on the floor in front of me, I silently cried as I gently brushed and pulled great handfuls of hair from her once thick and glorious crown. And then I shaved her head.

We both cried as she faced herself in the mirror for the first time, totally bald! Her reflection reminded her that this disease was real. Even the days with the chemotherapy still in progress, and with all the side effects she suffered, she still had good days when she could almost make herself, as well as me, forget it. But not when she had to face her reflection each morning in the mirror. No! That was a visible reminder that this was REAL!

"I beseech you to give her strength, and an extra measure of grace to deal with this," I silently prayed. "The world is cruel — the questions, the stares, the unwanted pity. I can't be there all the time to protect her from the world. I know you understand and You will be there for her." I had to trust Him, yet my heart was broken!

The next morning my son, Adam, went into the bathroom and was startled as he looked into the trash basket, through eyes still half asleep, and saw what he thought was an "animal." We all laughed as Andrew and I explained to him that what he saw was Joy's hair we had put there the night before. "Scared me half to death," he said. "I didn't have my contacts in, and I thought it was alive." It was the laugh I needed, and I thanked God for my son, the comic. Joy would hear about it later that day, and laugh too.

Weeks before, she and I had made a trip to the wig store, and so we were prepared when she arrived at my house a while later that morning to don her wig. You would have to understand our relationship in order to appreciate our humor. We laugh at the same stupid jokes, love off-the-wall humor, are crazy about Gary Larson's *Far Side*, make up our own endings to movies when the written ending isn't to our liking ... and, well ... we laughed so hard when she put that wig on. She made faces, and I combed it all crazy, and we were laughing hysterically. We eventually settled down, I combed it very nicely, and then she looked in the mirror.

"Does it look ... wiggy?" she asked very seriously. "I mean, say I'm walking down the street," she continued as she pranced into the kitchen, "and you see me, and don't know me. Would you say, 'She is wearing a wig! It looks like a wig'?"

"No," I said, trying without laughing at her antics to convince her. "I don't think it looks 'wiggy' at all. It looks very natural. It is almost the same color as your own hair; the style is just a little different." I rambled on, trying to encourage her to look at it in a positive light. "Trust me! I would definitely tell you if it didn't look good." I finally convinced her that it looked pretty real, after we placed a baseball cap on it, covering it up almost entirely!

"Yes!" she said, looking in the mirror. "The cap is what it needed!" I thanked God, for I knew that He cared as much about her feelings regarding the wig, as He did about anything else. That's only one of the many reasons I love Him so much!

Actually, as Joy got more comfortable with the wig, she also got more brave without it! Once when we were driving on I-495 on the way home from the doctor's office, we passed a car where several young boys were laughing, pointing at us, and making faces. All of a sudden she threw off her wig, and made a face back at them. The looks on their little faces were priceless! Never did they expect that! We rolled in laughter so hard that we actually had tears streaming down our cheeks, as we could only imagine the conversation that must have been taking place in that car. At other times she felt that the wig was too hot, and she would throw it across the room, or stick it in her gym bag at the softball field, to the astonishment of her teammates, not to mention the other team! That poor wig never did see a wig stand! Joy became anything but attached to it! It was at those times that I thanked God for her sense of humor, and for His obvious sense of humor as well!

After six months of chemotherapy and forty injections of the growth factor, we breathed a sigh of relief. Maybe this was it. Joy felt so normal, so alive, so healthy. Her blood counts, red as well as white, had remained good, and the doctor was very pleased with her progress. She had not even come close to having to be hospitalized! We were convinced that we had been given the "real" growth factor — and not the placebo — and that was the reason the white count had remained so high. We had prayed that she had been given the "real" medicine, and our prayers had been answered! We later found out to our amazement that she had been given the placebo! I had given her forty injections of saline solution! We didn't need the "real" thing because we had the "real" thing! God is the real thing, and He was all we needed. We were filled with praises to Him!

Chapter 7

Return With A Vengeance

July, 1992, marked one year since Joy's cancer had been diagnosed. Everything seemed to be going well. Her hair had grown back, and she was feeling pretty good. She was going to work every day, and we were convinced that she was cured. The only thing that bothered her was her back. Even six Motrin tablets didn't seem to relieve the pain.

I had begged her for a week to call the doctor, but as I have already told you, she is stubborn! She just kept putting it off. She finally agreed to call him only after the pain became so excruciating she could endure it no longer. She went in for her appointment, and x-rays were taken.

On July 20, just days before her thirty-sixth birthday, our worst fears were realized! The x-rays revealed a spot of cancer on her breastbone, her spine, and her left shoulder! I remember vividly the day we heard the news. The surgeon was to call her when she had gotten the results of the x-rays. We went from the doctor's office to my house to wait for the call. It finally came! I knew it wasn't good news as I heard her one-sided conversation with the surgeon.

"Yes. I understand, doctor. Yes, I'm all right, really I am. Yes, I will." And then as she hung up the phone and slowly turned around to face me, she was expressionless. She began walking through the house from room to room crying hysterically and screaming, "I don't believe this. It can't be true! It can't be happening again! I just don't understand it! I can't go through chemotherapy again! I just can't." She sobbed and screamed those same

32

haunting words over and over again! I let her scream and pace through the house until she was completely exhausted, and she literally fell onto the sofa. I placed my arms around her, she laid her head on my shoulder, and we both cried until we could cry no longer.

We didn't speak for what seemed like a very long time. It was then that we talked, and I prayed aloud for grace for yet another battle in this war. God's grace began working immediately in a way that I couldn't comprehend. We actually began laughing about the fact that we guessed He still had other "fun" experiences He wanted us to share together, and we supposed there were perhaps other lessons to be learned. I reminded her that He gives us nothing we cannot bear — nothing! But I have to admit that it was the first time I questioned in my heart, "Lord, how much more? Why, Lord, why?" She would need much more aggressive chemotherapy. She would lose her hair again! It had grown back now thicker than ever and, of all things, curly. She had complained at first about the curls until I reminded her that curly was better than bald — she had even gotten used to the curls, and now — she would lose it again. It didn't seem fair! I prayed for understanding, acceptance, but most of all for wisdom. I asked the Lord to forgive my doubt and make me strong! I needed to totally rely on His promise, "God is our refuge and strength ..." (Psalm 46:1).

Chapter 8

Chemo With A Twist

Joy's chemotherapy this time was to be for four weeks. We had to go to a subsidiary of the hospital called Intracare. It is an outpatient clinic with private hospital-type rooms, where patients can be monitored closely while taking this type of treatment. She would be in this facility for ten hours each session, while she received continuous chemotherapy. In order to do this, the doctor told her she would have to have a special port implanted in her body, just above the left breast. He told her that he had just received a new type of port that could be implanted completely under the skin. It was for active people who didn't like the inconvenience of an outer port. Of course, "active" certainly describes her, and since she had decided she WOULD continue to play sports (softball, volleyball, golf, and so forth), she opted to have the new port implanted. All her medications and chemotherapy could be given through that port, and it would no longer be necessary for a nurse to "find" a vein, a procedure which caused her a great deal of pain. She even accepted the fact that she would have to have "surgery" to put the port into place, because she knew in the long run, it would best suit her lifestyle. I thanked God again, for she had decided she would have the victory through Him. Her positive attitude had again been infectious to those around her and was a good medicine to us all.

The surgery to have the port implanted went very well. She had it done at the hospital as an outpatient. Although she dreads surgery, because she does not do well with the anesthesia, she did unusually well, and for that I thanked God. She was now ready to have her four-week course of "very aggressive" chemotherapy.

"Very aggressive," she said. "I thought the last I had was 'very aggressive.' How 'aggressive' can they get?"

"As 'aggressive' as it takes, dummy," I joked. Inside, I wondered myself how much more "aggressive" it could be, and I prayed once again for the strength of God's power.

Intracare was an interesting experience. We decided if we had to be stuck in a hospital room for ten hours, we would make the best of it … and that we did!! We took with us a VCR, movies we rented, a cooler filled with ice and cokes, bags of cookies, candy, chips, crackers, cups, plates, and so forth. We laughed and laughed as we carried our "equipment" into the building where we were met with looks of disbelief, which only made us laugh the harder. Ten hours is a mighty long time to stare at the walls or at each other, for even the best of friends can only do that for so long, so we took care of that in fine fashion! We "camped" out in style and made the best out of an otherwise dismal experience.

At the end of the ten hours, not only did we have to take back with us all of the paraphernalia we had brought in, but we also had to take a bag full of medicine, syringes (which by now I had mastered the use of), pages of instructions, a huge portable monitor to which she was hooked up (equipped with whistles and bells to alert us to possible problems), and a scale on which she was to weigh herself to make sure she wasn't retaining fluids (the pills to alleviate this potential problem were in our bag full of medicine). If we had stares when we came into the building, you can only imagine what we had when we left! We truly looked like "bag ladies" because, of course, we had to take it all to the car in one trip, according to "Miss I'm Not Going to Let Anyone Think That I Am Weak"! After all, she wouldn't want anyone to see how exhausted she really was! With what I had observed during the ordeal, I knew she had to be completely drained. I had only been sitting there for ten hours and I felt totally wiped out!

Once we made it to the car, which in and of itself was a monumental feat, we loaded everything in and drove home. Of course, she insisted on driving; she doesn't trust my driving! On the way home we laughed hysterically at how we must have looked as we left the office with things piled up, hung on, draped over, hanging out, tied on, etc. We joked about what would have happened if we had both fallen and dropped everything! That could have been a real possibility, but thankfully it didn't happen. We planned to be more organized the next time. However, I can assure you that no matter how hard we tried, we just couldn't manage to get everything to the car in one trip without great difficulty, and we "had to get it in one trip," so we struggled each time, and laughed each time, and planned to be more organized each time, and with the same end result! It became a joke with us as well as a challenge to her, to arrange and rearrange all the "stuff," for she never would accept defeat! But you know, it was those kinds of things that kept the humor in the midst of the nightmare, and I truly believe it helped keep us sane!

After we would arrive at home, we would fix dinner while joking about the events of the day, and for a while, she seemed to be perfectly fine. Then, after a couple of hours, the nausea and stomach cramps would start, and for a time we could not laugh at all. The reality of the cancer would set in once again. She laid on the sofa, and Jim, my mother and I would sit with her, each of us feeling very helpless. We all silently prayed as we tried to read, watch television, or talk quietly, trying to appear that everything was normal. You see, with Joy we had to carry on as if everything were "normal" or she felt like she was inconveniencing us or changing our plans. She never wanted to be a burden on anyone, let alone on us. And yet ... nothing felt "normal" to me at all. One day she was fiercely independent and full of life ... now she lay helpless and very much dependent. "Oh, Lord," I prayed, "let this pass if it be possible. Give her blessed sleep tonight. Give us all courage and wisdom as we minister to her."

After several long hours would pass, and I had administered anti-nausea medicine to her, kept cold cloths on her head, helped her with many trips to the bathroom where she experienced bouts of diarrhea and vomiting, she would then fall exhaustedly into bed and sleep would take over.

As Jim and I went to bed, it was then that I could talk and let go of my feelings through the cleansing of tears. With the wise counsel and encouragement of my husband, I would fall asleep with his arms around me knowing that he was praying for her as well as for strength for me. God had already given me that strength through his love and supportive understanding, and I thanked God again for my husband.

During those four weeks, she usually did very well through the night, once she had gotten to sleep. She never had to call me during the night to give her more anti-nausea medication, although she could have had it, and she was usually pretty perky the next morning when we would have to return to the Intracare facility. There they would remove all her tubes, whistles and bells, and she was set for yet another week. After those grueling four weeks were over, it became simply another waiting game — once again!

Chapter 9

My Life: Part One

The fall of 1992 brought new facets of stress into my life. Joy was progressing well. She was feeling stronger every day, and for that I was very thankful. It had been a long and painful summer, but it was over. Her treatments were going well, things looked good, and I felt refreshed as well as relieved.

Our boys had grown into young men; they were getting ready to leave home and start new chapters in their lives. I expected that; however, I was soon to find out that I was not at all prepared for the changes that I thought I was prepared for — not at all!

Our older son, Andrew, was engaged to be married in September to Julie, a lovely young woman he had been dating since his first year in college. I knew we would miss him terribly, but with Julie, we were gaining a daughter and God had answered our prayers above and beyond all we had hoped for.

She and Andrew had come from very different religious backgrounds and that, I admit, concerned us. Andrew had discussed his own concerns with his father and me. He desired above all that they be united in Christ. They even had a brief period of separation because Andrew knew that unless this happened, they could not have the marriage he knew was God's will for him.

They were both miserable during the separation. Therefore, Andrew decided if God wanted him to marry Julie, he would tell her his concern, and see what her reaction was. Unbeknownst to him, Julie had also decided to ask Andrew what his real reason was for their breakup.

The two of them had some pretty deep theological discussions in the weeks and months that followed, as Andrew explained to her his faith in Jesus Christ, and what it means to him, and how he wanted her to share in it with him.

Julie had been raised in a Catholic home with tremendous values and a belief in Jesus Christ, but not with the realization of how a personal relationship with Him could be the beginning of a lifestyle change that could not be equaled. She saw in Andrew, she told me later, what she had been wanting all her life. She desired to learn more about this "personal" relationship.

As their renewed relationship grew, it became clear to us all that Julie wanted for herself what Andrew also wanted for her. She has since admitted to me that at first she did want to please Andrew because she loved him so much, but she soon realized that the more she learned about Jesus Christ and a new life in Him, the more she knew she wanted this lifestyle for herself. She wanted Christ to be real to her.

They were engaged two years later and, as an engaged couple, attended a Family Life Seminar held in our area and sponsored by a tremendous Bible-believing church they now attend regularly. I felt peace in my heart, and we were excited about the marriage.

They were married September 26, 1992, by a wonderful Christian Army chaplain and our own pastor.

The morning of the wedding, Andrew came into our room, put his arms around me, and said, "I just wanted to hug you, and to tell you that I love you, but don't say anything, Mom." I hugged him hard as tears filled my eyes, and I simply told him that I loved him too, for I could see the tears welling up in his eyes also. We didn't need to say anything else. This was his way of letting me know he was now ready to start his own life, and with that I knew that the life we had provided, the values we had taught, and the faith we had led him to, were very precious to him, and it was the best "thank you" that any mother could have asked for. As I let go of him and he went to find his father, I thanked God for His priceless gift of our wonderful son and the realization that He had also now added to our family a blessed daughter as well. It is the hope of every Christian parent!

In the midst of all of Joy's treatments, the wedding was a most joyous time, even though I knew we would miss Andrew terribly. I was grateful that Joy was well enough to be a part of it, for the diversion had been such a great blessing. She had been so helpful and supportive to me with all of the wedding preparations, and she seemed like her old self. At the wedding, she looked absolutely like the picture of health, even if she did have to wear the hated wig! Physically, she seemed to be doing very well, and we all felt the "aggressive" chemotherapy must be working.

Although a wedding can be somewhat stressful, it is an exciting type of stress, and all too soon this phase of fall 1992 was over. However, nothing could have prepared me for the second phase!

You see, I must tell you about my life also, because when you make the choice to become an integral part of someone else's life, someone who has such deep needs, your life will be profoundly affected, as well as the lives of your family members. Don't even make a commitment of this magnitude unless you are willing to pay the price. And believe me, you will pay the price! I wouldn't change a thing about my commitment to Joy, and I thank God that He has allowed our family to minister to her. But cancer takes a tremendous toll on all the lives surrounding those whom it touches. It has taken a tremendous toll on my life, and when you factor in the everyday stress of handling a job and raising a family, as well as being the primary caregiver to an elderly parent, all of which I also consider to be a joy and a privilege, there were and still are times that I feel very much overwhelmed. It is then that God's promise to never give us more than we can bear (1 Corinthians 10:13) is such a comfort to me.

God surely has given me exceeding grace and strength to face all the pressures, for I could not have endured them without Him. But I was soon to find out that He would again give to me, just as liberally, the grace and strength that I would need to face yet another battle, and this time not for Joy but for me!

40

Chapter 10

My Life: Part Two

Our younger son, Adam, also left home the fall of 1992. He began his first year of college at Longwood College which is about three hours away from home. The "empty nest syndrome" was beginning to be very real to me. I was feeling useless! Adam was also having a hard time adjusting, even though his studies were going well, and he had a wonderful Christian roommate, Jeff, whom he already thought of as a brother. Some days he would call me four or five times. He would sound lonely, depressed and fearful, and would dissolve into tears. We tried to assure him that this was normal and that he would adjust. We really did believe that, although it was a difficult time for him as well as for us, it would pass quickly!

He then began to develop stomach problems; twice he had to be taken to the emergency room of the local hospital for treatment of a back injury that he had suffered when he was in high school. We still believed all these things were stress-related, and once more we took all the usual steps to try to help him work it out. We tried again to assure him that this would pass. We made trips to the college to visit, and we had him come home, even though we knew it was probably best for him not to come home or have us visit. I didn't know what was right or wrong. I just knew during those times he needed to see us. He seemed to live for the times we visited or made arrangements for him to come home.

He came home for Andrew and Julie's wedding and, of course, was very excited about being the "Best Man." He was in good spirits when he left to go back to school. But as soon as he returned, the same old pattern occurred again — the daily phone calls, the frantic sound in his voice, followed by the pep talks from his father and me. The situation seemed to be getting worse instead of better!

He told us he prayed about it all the time, but he just couldn't cope with the homesickness. He would tell me that he felt such an emptiness in his heart. That statement literally broke mine. We had just about decided to go get him and transfer him to a school near our home, for we had simply tried everything else. He would cry. I would cry.

Night after night as I lay in bed crying, Jim would comfort me and tell me that this would pass, and it would get better. But it soon became obvious to me, as the days and weeks passed with no change, that if Jim, who had always been able to "make things better," couldn't do it in all that time, then something was terribly wrong. I just didn't know what it was. We had prayed continually and tried everything possible, to no avail! We had finally decided that it was time to tell Adam that at the end of the semester he could transfer to a college near our home, if he really wanted to. We would tell him when he came home for Thanksgiving.

He got very sick again in November, two days before he was to come home for Thanksgiving, with what we thought was an intestinal virus. He followed our advice, staying off solid foods and drinking plenty of fluids. The day he was to leave campus to come home, he called us and told us that he felt even worse than before and was very weak and dizzy. He had even missed a class, something that he had never done! At our insistence, he went to the infirmary where he was told by the nurse that she also thought that what he had was an intestinal virus. He was to stay on clear liquids and drink plenty of fluids. That sounded familiar!

After convincing us that he could drive home, and only after his friend, Krista, seeing how sick he was, changed her plans in order to come with him, we decided to allow him to drive. God certainly was with Adam, because by the time he got home, he looked so weak that it frightened us. When he told us that he was still feeling dizzy, Jim thought that he might be experiencing an inner ear infection as well as something intestinal. Despite that, he told us that he actually felt hungry, so I fed him scrambled eggs and toast and pushed the fluids. He slept fairly well that night, and the next morning I made an appointment for him to see the doctor.

Before I could get him to the doctor's office, he began throwing up blood, and he collapsed on the bathroom floor. I got him to the car and drove him to the hospital. In looking back, I realize that I should never have done that. I should have called 911 and had him taken to the hospital by ambulance, where the EMTs would have immediately started an IV. By the time I got Adam to the emergency room, the doctor estimated that he had lost over fifty percent of the blood in his body! He was diagnosed as having a bleeding ulcer. He was quickly taken to the intensive care unit, and an endoscopy was performed to cauterize the ulcer in the hopes that the bleeding would be stopped. Thankfully, by that time, Jim arrived at the hospital! He had been in court some distance away when I got word to him of what I was doing, and I had prayed that God would keep him safe on the road, but bring him to us quickly!

I had never felt so helpless! Here was our eighteen-year-old, six-foot, 200-pound son, lying in the intensive care unit, with tubes stuck in his nose and throat, and as pale as I had ever seen anyone. We were very frightened at the prospect of losing him as the doctor told us of the seriousness of what had happened. The ulcer had been caused, he thought, by an anti-inflammatory Adam had been taking for his lower back problem. He told us that about eighteen percent of the population cannot take this type of medication, even for a short period of time, without serious complications. Adam didn't misuse the drug; he was just one of those eighteen percent. He had obviously been bleeding since the beginning of the school semester, but when he had been taken to the hospital for his back pain, the doctor had given him massive doses of the same medication he had been taking, unaware of the fact that it was further damaging Adam's stomach, and that had, of course, worsened the situation.

His doctor then informed us that because the bleeding was so severe, he had been unable to tell whether or not he had been successful with the cauterization. We would just have to wait and see. Also, there was a possibility that Adam would need a blood transfusion because of his massive blood loss. As the doctor explained this to Adam, big tears filled our son's usually lucent blue eyes, and he pleaded with us, "Please, no blood transfusion!" His father assured him that we would only consent to it if it became an absolute necessity. I simply could not speak for fear the wall of tears inside would crash through, and Adam would see my own fear. I just squeezed his hand, kissed him, and told him I loved him, and that everything was going to be okay.

I know the blood supply is supposed to be safe, but it was just another worry that neither an eighteen-year-old nor his parents needed, and so we prayed that his blood count would go up. We were thankful for a very conservative doctor who told Adam that because he was otherwise healthy, and in very good physical condition, there was an excellent chance the blood count would go up on its own. That seemed to relieve him, as well as his father and me. Of course, knowing the Great Physician was to be our greatest source of comfort!

We spent the next three days in and out of the intensive care unit. Jim and I as well as Andrew and Julie were in his room as often as we were allowed to be. Of course, Joy was also there to comfort and do whatever she could to make it easier on us. She loves Adam very much, and I knew she was praying for him just as earnestly as we were. I looked over at her often during those days and thanked God for answered prayers on her behalf over the past year. I was reminded again and again that God is faithful, and as I had trusted Him to take care of my friend, I had to trust Him then to take care of my precious son. She would remind me often that she knew firsthand of God's strength and power, for she was living proof of it! She had matured in the Lord so much over the last year, and that made my heart truly rejoice.

Our pastor was often there, praying with us, visiting with Adam, or just helping us to pass the time with conversation. Our family and church were in and out, praying with us, and encouraging and comforting. His grandmother was, of course, at home fervently praying and interceding for her youngest grandchild. Adam's friends were very anxious about him and called the house often. He is a very loved boy and we knew it. His college roommate and family called and reminded us of their prayers for him. What a blessing Jeff and his family had been to us in the short time we had known them. We are so thankful for them!

The first two days, Adam's blood counts went lower and lower, and it seemed as though a blood transfusion was inevitable. We continued to pray. His arms looked like pin cushions from all the blood tests. Each time we saw him, the first question was always the same, "Will I have to have a transfusion?" We kept encouraging him that the counts would go up, and we kept praying.

On Saturday the count began, ever so slowly, to go up! We were filled with praise to the Lord. Again, I stood amazed at the goodness of God, and again I was ashamed of my own doubt. I knew He understood and had forgiven me.

That evening, Adam was moved out of intensive care when another blood test revealed that the counts had gone up even further. On Monday, after a second endoscopy was performed to assure the doctor that the bleeding had, in fact, stopped, we took our son home. He had to have full rest for a week, and couldn't return to school until after the Christmas break, but he was home, and he was alive, and he was improving and — what marvelous answer to prayer! How thankful we were to our God!

Our Thanksgiving that year had certainly been different! We had made plans before Adam had gotten ill to continue our family tradition of going to our cabin in Luray, Virginia, for the weekend. Our plans had been changed, but we had never been so thankful! Thankful that Adam had gotten home from college before his condition had worsened, thankful for the excellent doctor, thankful that no transfusion had been necessary, thankful that our son was alive, and, of course, thankful that Joy was with us, and for all that He had done for her! What a special Thanksgiving season it was!

Adam's recovery was rapid, except that he tired easily. As he began to recover, he then began to worry about his exams. He didn't want to wait until he returned to school to take them. That would be a full month away!

God intervened in that situation also, and with the consent of his college professors and under the guidance of Adam's high school counselor, Mrs. Jody Blackwell, who was, and always has been, so wonderful and supportive to Adam, he took all of his exams at the high school the week before Christmas. He passed them all and ended up the semester with a 2.6 grade point average! We were elated, considering this very traumatic first semester.

In January, before Adam was to return to school, he spoke to us and to our pastor about being rebaptized. He said he felt that he had been so young when he had accepted the Lord and was baptized that he couldn't remember it. He wanted something to remember. He told the pastor that his salvation had meant so much more to him with all he had been through, and that he had felt closer to the Lord than ever before. The pastor arranged with us to have the service on the Sunday before Adam was to return to school.

When Adam entered the waters of baptism for that second time, everyone knew that this time was very, very special to him. Andrew and Julie were there, and Andrew played the piano for our service. I looked at both of our boys, and I was suddenly filled with overwhelming emotion! I thanked God for what our boys mean to me. I sometimes feel as though no children that were ever born are as loved as they are, and I realize that if every mother felt that way, the world would indeed be a different place, for that's the way God intended it to be! How very blessed I feel!

On the way home that afternoon, Jim turned to me and said, "I don't want this to sound irreverent, but as I looked at the boys today, I couldn't help thinking 'these are my beloved sons in whom I am well pleased'" (Matthew 3:17). I knew that he had been as overwhelmed as I had been, and we could only be filled with praise and thanks to God for His most precious blessings to us!

After learning from Adam's doctor that the medication that had caused the bleeding can also cause severe depression, we put the pieces of the puzzle together and realized that while Adam was indeed probably homesick that first semester at Longwood, the medication was most likely the main reason for the depression, which we had attributed to simply homesickness and stress.

Adam desired very much to return to school, and while he did call home rather frequently for a while, it was a dramatic change from the way he had been before. He adjusted beautifully and was a new person. I cannot tell you what a burden was lifted from me!

I thanked God for getting us through this crisis and for the strength of character He had shown us in our son.

Adam and I still fondly refer to his first semester as "The Great Depression," for at times we didn't know which one of us was the most depressed. Jim had to cope with both of us! When Adam used to call me every day, and sometimes several times a day, I would cry. And then when he got better and quit calling home so often, I would cry! Not, of course, because I was not greatly relieved that he was coping on his own, but because I realized how much I missed him. "The Great Depression" was now over, and God had gotten us through. We had grown closer to Him and closer together as a family. Praise God!

Chapter 11

The War Rages

During the winter months, with Adam's return to school, Andrew and Julie happily settled, and Joy feeling stronger (her hair growing back), I began feeling much less stress in my life. My mother's health, while up and down, was pretty good, and things seemed as normal as they could get with both of the boys gone. The house seemed LOUDLY quiet after the events of the last three months. I was beginning to adjust to the empty-nest syndrome even though I missed them both terribly. I thanked God for the extraordinary strength He had given to me and to Jim during that very stressful time. The strength I had prayed for Joy to receive, He had also provided to us.

With the spring of 1993, softball season was again in full swing at our church. Our team was doing very well due, of course, to our coach and star female player, you-know-who! The omega port Joy had been given was allowing her complete freedom to play ball without hindering her or slowing her up one step. She looked to be in great shape. She was on no medication, no chemotherapy and no pain! Or so I thought. She went periodically to have the port flushed out to keep it from becoming infected, but other than that, her hair was back ... yes, more curls galore ("Ugh!" according to her), and she didn't have any signs of the cancer at all. She seemingly went about her daily life with no problem. Life seemed great! Maybe, I thought, this was it. Maybe, just maybe, we are free of the CANCER! I prayed this to be true.

Then in July, again right before her (thirty-seventh) birthday, she began experiencing difficulty with her legs; however, she had said nothing to anyone, not even to me. One evening during a softball game, I suddenly realized that something was terribly wrong with her. She was on third base, and as she began running to homeplate, I saw her stumble as if her legs would not support her. It wasn't normal for her. She was called "OUT" at homeplate, and that definitely was not normal for her! I ran over to the bench, but at that time, with everyone around, she tried to brush it off. However, I could tell by the look in her eyes that she was in trouble. The whole team could tell!

After the game, she told me, through tears, that her legs had felt "squishy" and "rubbery," and she had felt like she had been running in slow motion. Then she confided that her legs had been feeling like that quite a lot in the past several days, but thinking it would go away, she had ignored it. She then told me she had been taking six to ten Motrin tablets before every game just so she could play! After I finished yelling at her for being so foolish and childish in not telling me this sooner, I told her that she had to go to see the doctor immediately! Even then, as frightened as she was, she wanted to wait until after softball season was over (only two more games) to call the doctor. I gave her a hundred reasons why she couldn't wait, but as I looked at her face, I knew she was thinking that this might be her last softball season — that is, as she had known softball, for as long as she could remember. With her pleading look, I made her promise only to coach those last two games, not to play, and to promise me, in turn, that she would let me know immediately if the pain worsened, and we would call the doctor whether or not the season was over!! She promised she would. I prayed again for wisdom as I asked the Lord to show me what to do. With Joy, you could only push so hard, and then you had to back off. I had to know when to back off and when to push harder. That took much wisdom!

The Lord took care of it, because two days later, when she came over to pick Adam up for the game, I realized by the way she was walking that the time had come to push harder. She could barely walk at all. Adam, who up until that time had not seen the most cruel effects of this disease as it destroys the body, looked very alarmed as he helped her to the sofa. I knew she must go to

49

the doctor right then! I took it upon myself without even asking her, and called the doctor, who advised us to bring her to his office immediately! Adam drove us to the doctor's office, and after the doctor's examination, he ordered her to be admitted to the hospital! An MRI discovered a tumor pressing against her spine and, if left alone and untreated, it would cause her legs to become paralyzed!

I will never forget the look on her face as the doctor gave her the results! It was her worst fear — to be paralyzed and in a wheelchair. She had often told me that she could take anything except that. ANYTHING!

"Don't you understand?" I told her. "God is gracious. You aren't too late to get treated, even though we had to practically drag you here," I said, trying to sound less fearful than I actually was. The doctor had told us that she would need at least ten days of radiation therapy, beginning that very day, to hopefully shrink the tumor. I instantly begin praying the radiation would do just that, and that she wouldn't lose heart.

One good thing about radiation is that you don't lose your hair, and you usually do not get sick. When she heard that, her spirits were again lifted, and she seemed resigned to taking the treatments, and the gloom began to lift from her face. However, when she explained to the radiologist who administered the treatment that we were to leave for the beach in about ten days, he told her he was not at all sure she would be finished with her therapy by that time! Her facial expression told it all! I have never before, even with all that she had been through, seen her so dejected. She lived for our vacations at the beach.

"All I had asked God for was the summer," she cried. "I have been asking Him all along to give me this summer." I knew that she was thinking that this might be her last summer, although she couldn't bear to say it. There was nothing I could say that helped. We would just have to pray and ask God to intervene, once again.

My heart ached as I thought of a vacation without her. The boys and Julie didn't want to even think about it when I told them of the possibility. It wouldn't be the same at all. I just prayed and prayed that God would allow her to go with us. "Oh, Lord," I asked, "please give us this summer together. She needs this so much, Lord. Give the doctor wisdom, and shorten the therapy time for her, if it is your will."

Only eight days later, I flipped on my answering machine and received that crazy message from her! God is so good!

Chapter 12

The Beach Blessing

With Joy's radiation treatment completed, the beach vacation that summer of 1993 was fantastic. We all had such a great time. As usual, God graciously gave us beautiful weather, and everyone, including Joy, was well.

I would watch her face as our boat skimmed across the bay — Jim at the helm, and she and I along for the ride. At times I saw tears brimming in her eyes as we watched the sunset or spotted the graceful osprey we searched for each time we were on the water. I knew there were some things about her disease that I could not be a part of. It was only between God and Joy. We all must deal with our own mortality at some point in our lives, and only God can give us the grace to face that; only He understands. I had my own tears as I studied her face and tried to feel the agony she must be going through. I prayed for God to keep giving her the grace to deal with it, for only He could.

Near the end of the week, she and Jim bought a used waverunner. What fun it was to have our own waverunner and not have to rent them. That had become an expensive form of amusement at $40 a half hour, and a half hour was never enough time! We purchased it two days before our vacation was over, but we sure made the best of it in that short amount of time. We named it the "Sandy Joy"! Adam and his college roommate, Jeff, who had spent the week with us, had a wonderful time riding it. The rest of us had fun too, when we could get them to take turns! However, we couldn't get Jim to take a ride. He says he is needed on shore to be able to bail us out of the water when, not if, we have a problem. We certainly had to be helped many times (especially Joy and me), so this was entirely a possibility. There was always next year for him, he would tell us! We vowed together, Joy and I, to make sure of that!

We took lots of pictures with our new "toy," and all too soon it was time to take it to the marina for winter storage. As Jim and the boys drove it away, I wondered if there would be rides next year — that is, like there had been this year, all of us together. The week had been very good, and it seemed like it had been our best beach vacation yet; I just didn't want it to be our "last" beach vacation.

I thanked God for wonderful family times with our special family and friends, and for this great vacation He had allowed us to have together. After all, I reasoned, Christ could return at any time, and we would all be together forever, and that would be okay too! The older I get, the more of life I experience, the more I realize just how awesome that will be!

Chapter 13

The Devastation

August 1993, and summer vacation was over. Once we were back home, it was time for Joy to go back to the doctor. It was on that visit that the doctor gave us the completely unexpected news! Joy must have a bone marrow transplant he told us, trying to sound as normal as possible.

"It is your only chance! Let me put it to you this way," he continued, knowing her love of sports, especially football. "We are backed up against the goal line, it's the fourth quarter, and we need a 'Hail Mary pass' because time is running out! We have read and studied all of your most recent x-rays, scans, and the results of your just completed radiation, and we feel there is just no other option!"

I could not look at her! I felt those hot tears choking me once again. My throat narrowed as if to close and squeeze the very breath out of my body! She seemed to understand what he had been saying, although the look on her face, when I dared to look, was that of shock. She did not cry or say much of anything as the doctor tried to be as positive as possible, explaining to us what she would need to do to prepare her body for the transplant, how successful transplants were, and so forth. I tried as best I could to remember everything, because I knew that she had not heard even half of what he had said. She was simply going through the motions in order to avoid displaying even a hint of the indescribable pain and agony she was feeling. She simply wanted to get it over with as soon as possible, in order to escape the stares and the pity written on the faces of the doctor and the nurses.

We talked with a nurse who set up the numerous appointments, tests, and so forth, that Joy would need before the transplant could take place. Joy smiled (although to this day I will never know how) as we finished, she made her usual jokes, and at long last, we left the office.

Neither of us spoke as we made our way to the car. I prayed for God to give me the wisdom to talk to her. Her disguise for the doctor and the nurses did not fool me at all. I knew her too well. I prayed for encouragement and peace. I prayed for strength and courage!

I was the first to speak as we began our twenty minute trip home. Although my mouth felt like it was full of cotton, I numbly explained what the doctor had said, and what we had just been told regarding this bone marrow transplant. She shook her head as if to tell me she wanted me to talk about it. I repeated their words, as if we hadn't heard them many times before, EXTREMELY AGGRESSIVE CHEMOTHERAPY! Prior to the transplant, she would be receiving EXTREMELY AGGRESSIVE CHEMOTHERAPY! She had already been subject to "aggressive chemotherapy," "very aggressive chemotherapy," and now she was to have "EXTREMELY AGGRESSIVE CHEMOTHER-APY!" Those words brought a chuckle from her, as we wondered out loud, what their next descriptive word might be. She motioned for me to continue.

That EXTREMELY AGGRESSIVE CHEMOTHERAPY, I reiterated, would take place four times during a several week period. In between those treatments, she was to have numerous tests, scans, x-rays and, something for diversion, a meeting with the head nurse of the bone marrow program at the hospital, and a "tour of the facility." (I remember thinking that sounded so strange, like it was a vacation spot or a country club one might be thinking of joining.) The nurses explained that Joy would be very busy with all of those things until the actual time of the transplant, so I told her I thought that part was good because it would leave her little time to let her mind dwell on the negative. After all of that, I continued, she would be allowed a short time of rest, and then the actual transplant would take place.

She let me ramble on, and all the while she didn't say a word, save the chuckle over the word describing the chemotherapy. When I was finished, her defenses dropped and she began to cry.

"I can't take the chemotherapy again! I just can't," she sobbed. "When will this be over? You don't understand how awful it really is. You try to understand, but unless you've been through it, you don't really."

I knew she was right, but I couldn't let her give up. "Yes, you can do it again!" I screamed at her, trying to sound so brave, and yet feeling myself falling apart inside. "God isn't finished with you yet. You have to let Him decide when you can no longer endure it. Every day you live is a day closer to a cure. Who are you to decide when enough is enough? We agreed to let Him have control, and now we must trust Him all the more." I had to say the words quickly before the tears that were inside choked me.

"I'm so scared," she now softly cried, sounding very vulnerable, and yet not defeated. "I'm so afraid. Doesn't God want me to be healed?"

I cried inside and asked the Lord, "How much more, Lord? How much more?" My heart broke for her as I tried to answer her question.

"He wants us to be more like Him with whatever it takes." That is all I could say. We both cried all the way home. It was the hardest test we had faced so far.

This latest turn of events was especially hard for Joy to accept, because only a few weeks before Pastor Trefry had conducted a special anointing service for her after prayer meeting one Wednesday evening. Jim and I, one of the other church elders, Charlie Worley, and his wife, Mary Rose, who had already been through her own battle with cancer and who is now in remission, were all a part of it. It was a beautiful service, and we all felt God's presence that evening. Now, with this crushing news, we had to trust Him with even more intensity.

Jim reminded Joy at supper one evening as we were discussing the transplant that this was perhaps God's way of providing a remission or a cure, and she had to accept His way and His timing no matter what it took to accomplish His will for her life.

"God doesn't always provide instant cures, although we know He certainly can," Jim quietly reminded her. "He also uses doctors and medicine to provide them too, if that is His plan." Isaiah 55:8 tells us: " 'For my thoughts are not your thoughts, neither are your ways my ways,' declares the Lord." She knew we had to trust Him.

Her spirits seemed to be lifted, and I truly believe that it was shortly after that conversation that she gave the cancer completely to God and asked Him to accomplish His work in her life in His own way, and in His own time — no matter whether or not this transplant would be God's cure, or whether or not she would ever be cured. She wanted to be more like Him, whatever it took!

Chapter 14

Thin Is In

CHEMOTHERAPY began yet AGAIN! How I grew to hate that word, and yet it was supposed to be killing the cancer cells, so for that, I was grateful.

"Will I lose my hair again?" she painfully asked Sunny, who would again be administering the chemotherapy.

"Well, probably," she said with a smile, knowing this was a big thing with Joy. "Although," she said with a lilt in her voice, "some people just have a thinning of the hair with this type of chemo."

"Okay!" Joy replied, with that familiar sparkle gleaming in her eyes. "I have very thick hair, so I think that it will just be thinner. Yes, I'm going for thinner! You think?" she added questioningly, while looking at me.

"Yeah," I said, noting her thick curls. "Let's just say thinner this time."

Sunny laughed and agreed with us, as she proceeded with the dreaded treatment. I prayed that she wouldn't lose her hair this time — that it would just be thinner, for it had meant so much to her.

During the next few weeks, she went for treatments, with blood counts taken on alternate weeks. Surprisingly, even though the chemotherapy was to be so aggressive, it wasn't too bad — bad enough, you understand, but not as bad as we had expected. And, praise God, no baldness — just thinning! This alone, not to mention the absence of the other side effects, made her very happy. I thanked the Lord again for the little things — the little things that meant so much to her!

Chapter 15

The Mothers — The Denial

During the months of August and September, 1993, much happened in both our lives. My mother developed congestive heart failure, and Joy's mother was hospitalized again for the return of her cancer. This time the cancer was affecting her brain! We spent much time helping each other out with visits to the hospital to see her mother, and multiple doctor's visits for my mother, in order to get her blood and heart rate regulated. Of course, all the while, Joy's treatments continued. It seemed for a while that all we heard from one day to the next was bad news.

To make matters worse, Joy's mother had been in the hospital only a few days when Joy received word by telephone that her father had died unexpectedly of a heart attack! Joy took the news with very little emotion. As she hung up the phone and turned to me, I noticed a lone tear in her eyes.

"Why am I shedding even one tear?" she asked. "He was never a father to me or a decent husband to my mother."

I saw deep into her heart that day and, without conversation, I realized the reason for the tear was just that — she had never had a father, and perhaps for the first time that realization hurt! God alone knew of the struggle she had with that part of her life, and He had closed the chapter! In a strange way, Joy actually seemed relieved. Not because he was dead, because to her knowledge, her father had never received Christ into his life, and for that, she was truly sorry. But relieved because he would never again have to be even a remote part of her life. She attended the funeral, and with that, it was over for her! I thanked God for His tender mercies and His compassion.

Opal had been permitted by her doctor to attend her husband's funeral, but soon afterwards had to return to the hospital. Her condition was very serious. The lymphoma had invaded her stomach, and it was discovered that she had developed a brain tumor as well. The silent killer had struck her body anew and with deadly force!

Fortunately, with medication, my mother began to respond to the blood thinners, and her condition stabilized after several weeks. I thanked the Lord that she needed no hospitalization and no heart surgery, both of which had been possibilities.

During those long weeks, I felt the "edge" closer and closer, and at times I found myself once again beginning to doubt! I felt as though nothing would ever be "normal" again. I could only imagine how Joy felt!

` She reacted by denial! Every time the doctor tried to tell her of the seriousness of her mother's situation, she would completely tune him out and would reach for anything at all to hold on to. All my attempts to get her to face the truth failed. She would get angry at me and refuse to discuss it at all! She always talked in terms of "when" my mother gets well — not "if." I had to give up and turn it over entirely to the Lord. I was at a total loss as to what to do.

"If I'm going to have to go through a bone marrow transplant, I need her to be there ... she has to be there ... she WILL BE THERE!" she screamed at me one day, and then, like a baby, she cried inconsolably! I knew that God would take care of helping her deal with it in His own time, and I just had to accept that.

It was during those times, the times that nothing I did or said seemed to help, that I would get the most angry. I would feel angry at Joy for not going to see the doctor when she first noticed the lump in her breast. I would get angry at the chemotherapy because it makes her so sick. And I admit, sometimes I even got angry at God! This disease has robbed me of my time, my energy, and my family. My life has changed because of it. I feel as though I, myself, have CANCER! I live with it every day, and I dream about it at night. It just didn't seem fair ... and then I would hear that "still, small voice" say, "I will never leave you nor forsake you" (Joshua 1:5). When I feel this anger, and I still do at times, God quiets my spirit with the reality of all my blessings, forgives my anger, and reminds me of his faithfulness, and I begin another day with renewed strength. It is then that I again give thanks to Him, for He is teaching me something valuable, something that He knows I need, something that can only be learned through trials and testing by fire! Something I need to help make me more like Him!

The week of September 20 was very traumatic. Joy's mother's condition was rapidly deteriorating, and every day brought more painful news. I watched as Joy made daily trips to the hospital even though she, herself, could barely hold her head up due to the effects of the treatments she was going through. This time she didn't have the vomiting or diarrhea, but instead the treatments rendered her very weak and extremely exhausted most of the time. The afternoon of September 21 brought a new dimension to the side effects of chemotherapy. Joy had done fairly well after her treatment on the previous day, but by the next afternoon, she was doubled over with intense pain in her chest. I called some of Joy's family to tell them that Joy could not make her usual trip to the hospital that evening because she was just too sick to leave my home. I don't think they understood at all. I felt a certain sadness for Joy, and for her family as well.

Because of the lack of communication in her family for many years, and because of Joy's desire not to let anyone feel sorry for her, I don't think many of them realized, or as yet realize, the scope of Joy's cancer, or the depth of her pain. She has always been perceived as the "strong" one, and she will never let them see her any other way. This has been, and continues to this day, to be the way it is. It has been her choice! Teri, her most beloved cousin, has been the only person in her family that I believe has understood, and she has been my contact point. It's certainly not that they don't care — I believe most of them care very much. It's just that some of them can't face the truth, so if they can remove themselves from the situation, it becomes easier for them. It is something that I have never understood, and never will. I am just thankful that God brought Joy and me together again after the long separation, in order that I might minister to her when she needed a friend and a family the most.

61

Joy spent Tuesday night and Wednesday night at our home because she was in a great deal of pain, and we didn't want her to be alone. An earlier call to the doctor had revealed that the exhaustion and intense chest pain were a normal reaction to the chemotherapy! All I could do was to pray for her, and go to her room periodically to check on her as she tried to get relief from the pain with the blessed gift of sleep. The tears in her eyes showed both fear and pain. Her look resembled that of a child who has briefly gotten lost from a mother. I knew her pain was a mixture of the side effects of the chemotherapy, and sorrow at the prospect of the death of her mother. I prayed for the nearness of the Lord and for sleep, and then when sleep would take over, I would go to my own room where sleep also comforted me.

Thursday morning, September 23, I called home from work to check on her. My mother, who had answered the phone, said, "Well, she is outside mowing the lawn!" You see, when she was well — she was WELL! Later on that morning when I called home again, Joy told me she had slept very well and was feeling great! Again, I marveled at the grace of the Lord, although I can't for the life of me understand why I was surprised, after all He had done!

Chapter 16

The Acceptance Of His Will

October, and Joy's mother was still critical. She had been in the hospital for eight weeks! Her stomach continued to swell from the tumor and fluid buildup; all attempts to shrink the tumor and the swelling failed. Her memory came and went from day to day, and then from moment to moment. She recognized and loved Joy one minute, and then in an instant she would forget and be unkind, even insulting. Joy would be terribly hurt even though she realized that the brain tumor was responsible. It had changed her mother's thought process. It was painful to see the tremendous toll it was taking on Joy, and most especially in her weakened condition!

It was after one particularly stressful visit with her mother that Joy finally admitted to me that she knew her mother was not going to recover unless God performed a miracle. She realized that Opal had already lived far longer than any of the doctors had ever imagined, considering the type of cancer she had. God had already performed that miracle, and they were both most grateful for the time He had given them together. The realization of this admission filled her eyes with tears, and my heart broke for her. It had been a long time coming, and a very agonizing thing for her to admit, but God accomplishes all things in His time.

"I'm sorry," she told me, "that I got so angry with you when you tried to make me understand how serious my mom's condition is. I just didn't want to face it." Several days before when I had tried again to talk to her about the reality of the situation, she had angrily screamed at me. "You have become a very negative person! Why must you always put a damper on everything!" I knew she didn't mean that. It was said out of hurt, fear and the reality of losing her mother. I had just prayed for the Lord to help her to accept the truth because I couldn't help her ... and He did. I praised Him for the barrier He had removed from between us, for now we could rationally discuss what before she had kept locked deep inside, for fear that even thinking about it would make it so. It was apparent that her mother was going to be taken from this earth soon. God was preparing Joy for it as only He can, and that was a burden lifted from me.

Joy continued her daily visits to see her mother, but with a different spirit and attitude. It didn't make it any easier for her to watch the suffering, but her understanding and acceptance of the situation helped her to cope. She tried to make her mother's last days as comfortable as possible, while constantly reminding her of her love. As sick as she was at times, Joy missed only one day visiting Opal in the hospital! Only God's strength enabled her to be strong, and she relied solely on Him for it. Truly it was an example of 2 Corinthians 12:9, 10: "My grace is sufficient for you, for my power is made perfect in weakness ... For when I am weak, then I am strong."

Chapter 17

A Change Of Plans

The week of October 10 was filled with more tests in preparation for Joy's bone marrow transplant. We were to know that week when it would be scheduled. I prayed for the cancer to be silenced in order to give her body a chance to receive the transplant. She was in pain again — coughing, feeling very tired, and very, very discouraged, especially with her mother's condition continuing to worsen day by day. "We need you more than ever, Lord," I prayed. "Much more ... she is exhausted! And, Lord, so am I!"

On October 15 she had a doctor's appointment, and we were to be given the date for the transplant. I remember thinking that I should have gone with her to her doctor's appointment that day because she never thinks to ask questions, and she never really hears everything that she is told. I have always been there to take notes and to hear what she misses. But I had missed so much work that when I thought she could handle a test or an appointment on her own, I felt like I had to go to work and save my leave in order to be able to use it when she really needed me the most.

I called her when I got to the office to remind her to tell the doctor about her persistent cough. "Okay. Okay!" she said, sounding a little annoyed at my "motherly" tone. She agreed to call me after her appointment, and after she had gotten to work.

Yes! She worked every day that she possibly could work. Phyllis, her supervisor, was aware of the situation, and often called me to get the latest information from the doctors' reports or just to talk. Joy is really loved at the NBC studios where she has worked for the past eighteen years. She is a loyal and faithful employee and very hard working, and Phyllis is very concerned and most supportive. She tries to monitor Joy to try to keep her from pushing herself at her job, although she realizes that for Joy, working is probably good medicine. We have become friends over these past few years, and I thank God for her.

When Joy finally called me later on that morning, I wasn't in the least prepared for the report. Oddly enough, she didn't seem upset at all! The bone marrow transplant had been canceled because the bone marrow aspiration, which had been performed a few days earlier, revealed that too many cancer cells had invaded her bones! I tried my best not to sound terrified as she continued to tell me that the doctor was going to try a "stem cell transplant" instead.

"What is that?" I said, feeling very guilty that I had not gone to the doctor's office with her.

"Well," she replied, while obviously munching on something, and sounding what one might call "chipper," "it's almost like a bone marrow transplant except it isn't nearly as painful, and I won't have to spend as long in the hospital. Isn't that just terrific?"

I didn't know what to say. I felt lost for words. How could the disease have traveled to her bones so fast? It seemed as if her body had been constantly full of chemotherapy! I tried not to sound fearful, as I continued to question her.

"Cheer up," she quipped, knowing by the sound of my voice that I was apprehensive, to say the least. "This will be good! Honest! The doctor seemed very optimistic!"

With that cheerful admonition, she hung up, only after I told her I wanted to be with her when she went for her next appointment, at which time the new procedure was to be discussed.

I was left with a feeling of complete discouragement. What did this really mean? She only hears what she wants to hear. I am thankful that she is always so positive, but she also tends to ignore warnings and instructions. Sometimes what you don't want to know, or choose not to do, can hurt you! I had seen that proven out several times during the past two years that we had been engaged in this war. I regretted again not having been with her. I felt very guilty!

Jim called me later that morning and asked me to meet him for lunch, a luxury that I rarely get in my job. It couldn't have come at a more perfect time, because I didn't think I could concentrate on my job any longer. As we hurriedly ate a sandwich and I relayed to him the contents of Joy's phone call, he reminded me that if we are supposed to live each day as if it were our last, because none of us are guaranteed even our next breath, then Joy is certainly doing exactly that! And if we were going to help her through this, we had to do likewise, living one day at a time and trusting Him moment by moment!

"You have to adopt her same attitude," he gently scolded. "That is, if you are to help her at all. Maybe we can plan some small trips or something in the spring, to give her things to look forward to. You have to be focused in order to keep her focused."

That short but sweet conversation was all that I needed to hear. I thanked God for my husband as I went back to work with a new attitude and God's amazing strength once again pulsing through my veins!

Chapter 18

Peace That Transcends All Understanding

Throughout the entire next week, Opal's condition deteriorated. By Friday, October 22, her blood pressure was almost nonexistent. I prayed all week that the Lord would take her home if she were not to be healed. Joy was both physically and emotionally drained.

Friday evening I accompanied her to the hospital. Her mother had worsened drastically since the morning. I prayed as I watched her life slowly slipping away. I prayed that He would take her. I cried as I heard Joy telling her mother, through agonizing sobs, that she loved her, and I listened to her heartbreaking words. "I'll be okay, Mama, honest I will. It's okay." There was nothing left to do except to let God take her in His time.

Pastor Trefry came in and had prayer for Opal and her family as we all held hands around her bed. He prayed for God's mercy and His grace. My heart was very heavy with grief! I couldn't stand to see Joy watching her mother's obvious agony during these last few days, knowing that the same disease that was soon to claim her mother was invading her own body and trying to claim her life as well. She needed all the strength she had to fight her own battle!

Very early the next morning, Opal's battle ended, and God took her home. The look on her face now was that of peace and serenity. Joy was able to thank God for taking her mother home for she had accepted His will. She knew she would miss her mother terribly, and that things would not ever be the same, but she couldn't keep her, knowing she was suffering. Oh, the grace of God, how great He is!

Opal was buried the following Tuesday, but we knew that her soul was with the Lord. I prayed for strength for Joy to get through this so-called civilized process known as a funeral. It was, for many who attended, and who had no hope, a traumatic and grief-filled day. It wasn't the type of service that Joy would have planned, if it had been left up to her. She told me later of her own plans for a service — a service filled with praise and glory to Jesus Christ. Not sad and depressing.

"Please promise me that my funeral will be glorifying to Jesus Christ, and joyous, not like this one was," she pleaded to me with tears streaming down her face. "I mean if God doesn't choose to heal me ... Promise?"

"I promise," I said, as I fought back bitter tears.

On our way back home from the funeral, we discussed death and dying and the events of the day. She said that she found herself actually rejoicing through the service that the Lord had taken her mom, for she knew that her mom was now enjoying a new life, free from cancer and pain. Her mother's courage and strength up until the end had made her more determined than ever to fight the battle. She revealed that for more than a week before her mother died, she had been praying that the Lord would take her home quickly, if He did not choose to heal her. I marveled that God had answered yet another prayer, for we had both been praying for the same thing, and I had been afraid to reveal that to her earlier. I had seen God accomplish in my friend's life a maturity and a wisdom that only He could have, and her face revealed the peace that the world could not understand — truly, a "peace which transcends all understanding" (Philippians 4:7)!

Chapter 19

A New Home

Knowing that only time and God's comfort could heal the pain of her mother's death, I now prayed solely for Joy and the ordeal yet before her. She had been having pain in her legs again and constant pain in her back. Again, with much persistence from me, her nemesis, she had gone to see the doctor on the day before her mother's funeral. After his initial exam, it was decided that she would need yet another MRI to reassess her condition. "Oh, Lord," I earnestly prayed, "let us have a little good news. She has been through so much lately. She needs a little sunshine ... Yet, 'my grace is sufficient ...' " (2 Corinthians 12:9).

She went in for the MRI two days after the funeral, and we went the following day to get the results. When God sent a little sunshine, He also sent a rainbow to go along with it! The MRI showed the cancer in her back was somewhat improved, and a second bone marrow aspiration showed no cancer cells in the bone marrow itself! The sun broke through the clouds as we were driving home from the doctor's office, and we thanked Him again for His never-failing love. We needed to have some encouragement, and He had supplied it abundantly. Our hearts were filled with gratitude. We began to pray for wisdom for the doctor and for the success of the stem cell transplant.

The weather stayed lovely for the next two days as we moved Joy into an apartment which was located much closer to our home. There were tears in her eyes as we drove away from the home she had shared with her mother. So many memories were there, and it was hard for her to face yet another reminder that this new chapter in her life would not include her mother. I reminded her that Opal would be very happy knowing that she was in a nice apartment in a safe neighborhood while being closer to us and our church. I could now easily care for her when she came home from the hospital. Joy was silent for a while, and I sat by quietly, allowing her time to sort out her own thoughts.

By the time we drove up to her new apartment, we were laughing as we realized how funny we must have looked in her small car with boxes piled up to the roof and with only our heads showing! We laughed at Jim as he "struggled" to back the truck up to the doorway while pretending he couldn't stop it!

Jim, Andrew, and several men from our church began unloading the truck. As Joy and I unpacked the boxes and began our usual slapstick antics, I realized this was where God wanted her to be. It just felt right for her. She was already beginning to adjust.

We spent the next few days fixing up her place with security locks, curtains, pictures, and, of course, her coffeemaker. It was beginning to look like a home. We were very exhausted, but it was a good kind of exhaustion because she was now where she needed to be, and the transition had been made quickly and smoothly with all of us working together.

When we left her to spend her first night alone since her mother's funeral, she seemed a bit apprehensive. It was the first time she had been completely on her own since she had left for college. But I knew and she knew that she would never truly be alone, for the Comforter was there … always there, and she would be just fine!

Chapter 20

The New Plan Revealed

Joy's cough was relentless! She just couldn't shake it; the medicine she had been given just didn't seem to be working at all. Her plans to go back to work November 8 were not carried through. She called me that morning. I talked her into staying in bed, and I insisted that she call the doctor once again.

"I feel just terrible, and my cough is worse than ever!" she complained. "I want to go to work, but I just don't think I can."

For Joy to admit she felt too sick to go to work, I knew she must have felt dreadful. I reminded her that she had to be extra cautious now with the transplant close at hand. It didn't take much persuasion this time; she agreed to call the doctor. I prayed fervently for the Lord to touch her body and make the way clear for the transplant. She needed to be as strong as possible. I was seeing something in her that I had never seen before, and it alarmed me. I saw her body unable to rebound. In all the years I had known Joy, she had never been sick. She had never missed work because of illness, never missed church; nothing had stopped her. Nothing! That is, until now! It was just another facet of the devastation of this disease. Just when she would begin to feel good, it would attack her body in yet another way, reminding her that it was still present. Even the "cure," the chemotherapy, attacks and weakens the heart and the lungs, causing shortness of breath and weakness. I had seen her once tireless body now showing signs of weakness and deterioration, not only from the cancer itself, but from the "cure" as well! I felt anger, frustration, pain and sorrow and.... "Help me, Lord," I prayed. "I feel powerless and afraid. I need your strength."

By Wednesday, November 10, with new medication, she could no longer be persuaded to stay in bed. She sounded better and perkier, and I actually thought it would be best, if she felt like it, for her to go back to work. She had missed so much work over the past several weeks, and with the knowledge that she would be missing much more very soon, she was anxious to get back.

The new medication continued to keep her cough under control, and by Friday, when I went with her to the hospital to see the doctor, she actually seemed like her old self.

Linda, the nurse in charge of the transplant program at the hospital (we called her Morticia, the Vampire), explained why she had to draw from Joy ten vials of blood, after which the doctor began to recount why he would be performing a stem cell transplant in lieu of a bone marrow transplant. All of this Joy took in stride, while maintaining her sense of humor. Linda took an instant liking to her, and, of course, her doctor, knowing her very well by now, was still impressed with her spunk and spirit. He tried to describe the transplant to us as simply as he possibly could.

The stem cell transplant is a procedure similar to that of a bone marrow transplant. It involves bringing to the blood's surface the yet immature blood stem cells (which are produced in the bone marrow), skimming the cells off the surface of the blood, processing and purifying them, then storing them. The body is then subjected to four days of high doses of chemotherapy, hopefully killing all cancer cells that may be present. The purified blood stem cells are then reintroduced into the body where they begin to produce new (keep praying), cancer-free cells.

Sounded simple enough, but when we were told what had to happen before any of that could take place, we couldn't believe it! For six days, I had to give her not one, but now TWO shots of the growth factor. The purpose of the growth factor is to bring the immature blood stem cells from the bone marrow to the surface of the blood. After those six days, she would go the hospital for several hours a day, during a four-day period, and be hooked up to a machine, similar to a kidney dialysis machine. This machine skims off the immature blood stem cells from the surface of the blood, after which they were to be purified and frozen until needed.

To prepare her body for the re-infusion of these cells, she would first be hospitalized, and then be subjected to four days of "mega aggressive" (our new term) doses of chemotherapy.

Unfortunately, this type of chemotherapy destroys your entire immune system, while also attempting to destroy all the cancer cells. Therefore particular care is taken so as not to expose the patient to infection. All precautions are taken to insure this ... hand washing, masks, gloves, and, of course, a private hospital room. After the four days of chemotherapy, she would have two days of rest, and then the purified blood stem cells would be returned to her body where they should begin to grow and start producing (keep on praying) healthy blood cells.

"In other words," I said, trying to lighten the otherwise heavy, heavy conversation, "you're stripped of all your ability to fight infection, taken to the brink of death, and just before you go over the edge as you gasp your last breath, you are given the new blood stem cells, and you are returned to the land of the living! Is that just about it?"

"That's just about the way it is," Linda replied through laughter. Joy looked at me and I looked at her, with our usual "you've got to be kidding" looks, and we said almost simultaneously, "How many of these procedures have you all done?"

Without blinking an eye, she answered, "One."

"One! As in one, two!" Joy said, looking at me in disbelief.

"Well," Linda continued, undaunted, "it has been done hundreds of times in other centers across the United States, but just not here ... yet. But don't worry! You will be just fine. Trust me!"

This, from a gal who had just taken ten vials of blood from my friend! We nervously laughed, but then we both began asking questions, questions, and more questions, until by the time we were ready to go home, we were actually pretty comfortable with the whole idea. You see, the One we "trusted" was the Lord Jesus Christ, and that made all the difference! We knew He was in charge and had been since the whole ordeal had started.

We prayed together on our way home, committing the doctors and the nurses to Him. With one exception, that of having to have yet another port "surgically" placed in her chest for purposes of the transplant, Joy seemed to be in extremely high spirits.

"What do you know? They have only performed one such procedure!" she quipped. "God is certainly testing us with this one." But even that was said with a calmness and a peace that only comes from the source of power that she was plugged into, and it was very evident!

The next week was filled with tests, tests, and more tests to prepare her body for this relatively new (and thought to be experimental by some experts) procedure. While her body was being prepared, I was praying that the Lord would prepare her mind and her heart as well.

We spent the week of November 8 (in between tests) trying to do our Christmas shopping. I went to work, she would go to have one of her many tests, then she would pick me up after work, and we would go to the mall. Last year, we had purchased all of our presents, and even had them wrapped, before Thanksgiving, and we determined to do the same thing again. We had two weeks before Thanksgiving in order to do it, and so we wasted no time at all.

Christmas! The most joyous time of the year for all of us, and yet I saw the pain on her face as we began our first shopping spree.

"I miss my mom so much just now," she softly cried, as I got into the car. "Christmas won't be the same this year without her."

I didn't know what to say, so I just grabbed her hand and we didn't speak for a while. I just silently prayed for God's peace and healing, but I knew it would take time. When we did talk, we both agreed that this Christmas had taken on an even deeper meaning for her as well as for me. We realized and appreciated even more than ever before the value of life, and what is really important. Christ came into the world to give us the greatest gift of all times, and He paid the ultimate price for it. And yet we, as Christians, take it for granted until, faced with our own mortality, we are made to wonder what we have done to deserve this gift, and what impact, if any, we have made on the world for Him!

We flew through the mall with reckless abandon, as we made purchase after purchase, and trip after trip to the car, depositing our bags and boxes. For a while she seemed like her old self, as we went on with our usual foolishness and laughter. However, before long, I began to notice that she needed to sit down more often, and although I didn't question her, I knew the ordeal was physically draining on her once tireless body. At my insistence, we abruptly put a halt to our shopping for the day, and I literally dragged her to the car.

Later that evening, I mentioned to Jim that I could see more and more the toll the cancer was taking on her body. He also had noticed that her usual unstoppable efforts were now greatly slowed, and her stamina was diminished. We had both seen it before our very eyes, and it was frightening! We continued to pray for strength for her, and the grueling ordeal yet to come. We needed to recall: "It is God who arms me with strength and makes my way perfect" (2 Samuel 22:33).

Chapter 21

We Give Thanks Once Again

My heart felt very heavy as I contemplated our annual trip to the mountain for Thanksgiving. I needed much wisdom because I was to begin giving Joy the growth factor shots ... again! How I had grown to hate — literally hate — giving those shots! I had to keep in mind that they were helping to keep her white cell count up, and that was very important, especially this time. The day before Thanksgiving, she picked the injections up at the doctor's office and came to my school for her first injection. The shot seemed unusually painful for her, and tears welled up in her eyes and streamed down her face. I felt hot tears stinging my eyes as well, and I wondered how I could do this not for six days, but, with a change in doctor's orders, now for ten days, twice a day! She rested in my office for about fifteen minutes after the injection, and then went off with Adam to do some errands before we were to leave, later that evening, for the mountain.

I arrived home from work early that afternoon and immediately received a call from Adam telling me that Joy was experiencing severe bone pain, and that they were on their way home. I could tell in Adam's voice that he was very panicked! I met them as they drove up to the house, and the two of us had to practically carry her into the house, because she could not walk. I immediately called the doctor and was somewhat relieved to learn that while this was very painful, it was not unusual. He told me to give her three Advil, two Tylenol with codeine, and two Benadryl tablets one hour before the next injection was due, to see if the pain was alleviated. She laughed, through tears, as I relayed that message to her.

"Well, maybe the object is to knock me out so I won't be able to feel the pain," she said. We released our tension through laughter, and I praised God that her severe reaction to the injection had not been abnormal.

"Oh, Lord," I prayed, "thank you for your unfailing love and the constant reminder through her laughter that You are in control."

I immediately telephoned Jim, and we questioned the wisdom of going to the mountain for the entire holiday weekend, due to her violent reaction to that first injection. The doctor had approved her going with us, but we felt so responsible! We decided to wait and make a final decision later on in the day.

Even the mere mention of our not going brought forth a cry that far surpassed the cry from the pain of the injection!

"I can go," she yelled! "The doctor told you it was okay."

"I know he did," I calmly replied. "But we may not be able to go to the mountain until after Thanksgiving day anyway because Jim just told me when I talked to him that he has too much work backing up at the office. Maybe we will have Thanksgiving dinner here, and then spend the rest of the weekend up there. That wouldn't be so bad would it?" I quickly added, before she could object too much! "We could still stay Friday and Saturday." Jim and I had decided this plan would make it seem like shortening the trip was in Jim's best interest and would be a way of hiding our real concern.

"Well," she replied, seeming to buy into the plan, "you do whatever is the best for him, but don't let me be a concern because I can go, and I feel really good now. I want to go no matter how short the stay."

She really did look much better, and it was obvious that the pain she had, though severe, was short-lived.

Joy dearly loves to go to our cabin in Luray, Virginia. The pace of living is very much different from that of Northern Virginia. The people are very friendly and laid back, and the scenery is some of the most beautiful in the United States. We've made few trips there that we haven't seen deer, wild turkey, foxes, and even bear. Our cabin overlooks the Blue Ridge Mountain range, and the Shenandoah River. The sunrises are spectacular. The cabin has particular meaning to us because we built it ourselves. We helped clear the building site and planned and built the house. The boys, even though very young at the time, helped put up walls, paint and finish it. They spent many, many hours making trails through the woods on which they would ride the All Terrain Vehicle we bought for them. They picked berries which were made into delicious pies and cobblers, and then, when they were older, learned how to drive a car on the remote back roads surrounding our property. They cultured from their father respect for guns and how to use them. Everything about that property reminds me of family and sharing, caring and loving. It was an experience that can never be replaced, and I will cherish the memories forever.

Joy, too, has wonderful memories of great times there, and I knew she didn't want to miss an opportunity to make another memory. Her particular fancy is the local gun shop. The owner is very friendly, and she, Jim and the boys have purchased several guns from him over the years. The shop is usually filled with "real" hunters. Our only "game" are cans, plastic bottles or paper targets. I'm sure they recognize us as city slickers. A trip to that shop is always an adventure. Joy's Christmas presents for the boys that year and my Christmas present to Jim were to be western boots. We had purchased them so that they would, as she put it, "Look like real residents."

Yes, praise God, we did go to the mountain for the entire Thanksgiving weekend! The second injection I gave her later on that evening, after the trio of pain killers took effect, went much better than the morning dose. She was sleepy, obviously, but the bone pain was GREATLY reduced. There was much to be thankful for! Adam was well this year (what a difference from last year), and God had answered so many prayers for Joy that we couldn't help but be filled with praise to God for His faithfulness.

Our last two Thanksgivings had been out of the "norm," but we had hearts that were overflowing with praises to our Lord and Savior, Jesus Christ!

Chapter 22

It's A Woman Thing

The injections were continued, and with each one I administered, I felt pain. The only thing that helped was the knowledge that I was playing an integral part in the fight to save her life, and it was something that I could do to keep myself from feeling so utterly helpless. I realized that she needed me and, in turn, the thought of losing her made me realize that I also needed her. God has given us a friendship that is very precious, and I didn't want to lose it.

Women form very special bonds and friendships that I don't think men quite understand. They don't form the same type of relationships with each other. I think God made women unique in that way. Men joke about women going to the bathroom in groups, or having to call each other to find out what the other is wearing to dinner, and so forth. We borrow clothes from each other, and we do talk on the telephone for long periods of time about everything or nothing. But you will find few women who don't have a special friend with whom they form that close bond, and when that bond includes Jesus Christ, it is indeed unique! Some men do not accept this at all. Jim, while perhaps not fully understanding, accepts this as a part of life. He knows that he is truly my best friend, next to the Lord, but Joy is my best girlfriend.

I once knew a woman whose husband forbid her to have another woman as a friend. I felt very sorry for her as she confided to me how she lived her life in fear of her husband! No, not fear of physical abuse, but emotional abuse. She had met another woman at her church and they had become friends. She longed to have this woman's company because, since she did not work outside of the home, she had no other contact with people. Her husband had forbidden her to have a job or to even learn to drive a car. When their children grew up and left home, she was truly lonely. She could not make phone calls during the day because he told her he needed to be able to reach her at any time. She couldn't leave the house because he told her he may need her. Oh, she could go to church every time the doors were open, because he wanted the church to see how much he loved the Lord! Little did they know what emotional trauma he was inflicting upon his wife. Her only outlet became the grocery store! She was able to persuade her husband to let her go the grocery store once a week with her friend. Of course, her time there was limited by him, but it was time she had with her cherished friend. She would tearfully tell me how much she looked forward to her once-a-week excursion to the grocery store. It was her special place where she could spend time with her friend, and share her thoughts, concerns and prayer requests. Here was a woman who loved, of all things, the grocery store! Because, you see, to her, it was so much more. She was so thankful to God for that small pleasure. I felt so ashamed at the way I take so many things in my marriage for granted. Of all the household chores, I hate the grocery store more than any of them, and for years Jim has been doing all of the grocery shopping for us. And here was a woman who loved the grocery store and was thankful to God that her husband had "allowed" her to go there!

We have always had a partnership in our marriage. Jim is the head of our household, but I feel equal. I never have to be afraid to express an opinion or an idea, and he will be the first to tell you that sometimes I have strong opinions. Yet, I have never felt that I was not valuable to our home. I thank God for Jim every day of my life, but talking to that woman made me so much more aware of God's blessings. I've lost contact with her over the years, but I can't help wondering when her husband will become the "real" man of the house and let Christ become the head; when he will let God control his life so he can release the control he has over his wife, and she can blossom and become the woman God wants her to be. She has great potential, and he is missing so much in life because he won't allow her to grow. He is not getting God's best for himself nor for his wife. I pray he will be open to the Lord's leading in his life before it is too late!

The friendship between Joy and me is an important part of my life. It has become an important part of Jim's life as well. He has accepted my role in her life during the past few years with support and love. I realize that few men could have done that. I will be eternally grateful to him for his understanding, his compassion and his love. He is God's greatest treasure to me!

Chapter 23

Phase One Of The New Battle

The day arrived for Joy's second port to be put into place. We arrived at the hospital at 4:00 p.m., November 29, with surgery scheduled to start at 6:00. After she registered, we had a little time to just sit and talk. She was very apprehensive, as she always is before surgery, due to problems she has encountered with anesthesia. Tears splashed down her cheeks, as she asked me to pray for her right then and there, before she had to be taken to the operating room. I prayed for her and for wisdom for the doctor. She looked so vulnerable at that moment, so dependent. I hugged her hard as the nurse came to take her away. "Oh, Lord," I cried, "may your peace encompass her. May she feel your presence."

The two-and-one-half hour wait seemed like an eternity, as I sat in the lobby waiting for my name to be called telling me that it was over, and I could take her home. The hospital staff was busily decorating the hospital for Christmas. As I sat there and watched all the hustle and bustle, I couldn't help but question how everyone could go about their lives as if everything were normal, when for us, nothing was normal at all. It didn't seem right. It didn't seem right at all! And, yes, I didn't think it was especially fair! But life does go on and I know we have to accept what God has for us, and remember that He is in control. If we have not life in Him, we have no life at all! And I know I'd rather have Him in my life, no matter where He leads, than to have everything "normal" and not have Him. I know that Joy feels that very same way. She would choose life with cancer, rather than a cancer-free body without Christ in her life. With Christ in one's life, one can face anything,

83

but without Him, there is no hope at all, for "real" life far exceeds our life here on this earth. Reflecting on this wonderful truth gives me real peace and puts everything back into perspective again.

As I sat back and watched the activity of the staff, I wondered how many of them really knew the full impact of that "first" Christmas, or the true value and price that was paid for God's most precious gift to the world, and how acceptance of that gift can forever change a life!

At 7:15, I heard my name called. After the doctor reassured me that everything went well — they just got a late start — I was called to the recovery room, where that ever-present smile greeted me as I came through the door.

"I'm so glad you were here with me," she rambled on and on while running her sentences together. "It was actually pretty rough because my veins, of course, do not cooperate, but I just knew you were praying for me and waiting ... I'm so sorry it took so long ... Did it seem like a long time?"

When she came up for air, I replied sarcastically, but with a grin, "Oh no! Not at all! Two and one-half hours is not a long time! I just thought they had lost you or you had decided to skip the whole thing and go on a vacation or something! Not to worry though — the hospital staff kept me entertained by putting up the Christmas decorations in the lobby. No wonder your hospital bills are enormous! There had to be at least thirty staff ... and no, they were not volunteers ... down there to decorate a couple of trees and put up a few wreaths!"

We giggled quietly trying to keep our voices down so the nurses would not hear us. I was so thankful to God that she seemed to be doing so well. Her laughter was such a great blessing to me. After about an hour in the recovery room, she was ready to go home, and I went to the garage to get the car. I picked her up at the door of the hospital, but as soon as we were out of the driveway, she insisted on driving home!

"I don't trust your driving after dark, and I am perfectly fine!" she succinctly stated.

I do have problems with astigmatism, and my night driving is affected, but I knew I could certainly drive home and I tried to convince her of that. I knew it would be to no avail, so I pulled over to the side of the road. She slipped behind the wheel, laughed her "I got my way again" laugh, and we drove away.

As we neared home, she reached over and squeezed my hand. "It meant so much to me that you were there," she said through tears, her stoic mask slipping away for a few brief moments. "I was really scared, and just knowing that you were there helped so much. You'll never know what your friendship means to me!"

I reminded her, through tears of my own, that she would have been there for me, and I thanked God that we had gotten through the first phase of this battle.

She cried that night as I gave her the scheduled injection of the growth factor. In fact, we both cried. The emotions were just too much to keep under control any longer, and it was indeed time for a good, long cry!

"I wish this whole thing were just over with!" she said through bitter tears. "I'm so tired of it all!"

I tried to console her as best I could, and we both cried our eyes out! But before too long, as only we can, we were both laughing and giggling like two schoolgirls. I thanked God for His gift of laughter ... what great medicine it had been for us! What great truth is found in Proverbs 17:22: "A cheerful heart is good medicine...."

Chapter 24

Phase Two With A Little Angel

The next day, November 30, Joy reported to the hospital to have the stem cell withdrawal. She was to have it done as an outpatient. Because of the nature of the procedure, and because it had been fully explained to her beforehand, she wasn't the least bit apprehensive. She wanted to go by herself; she assured me she would be okay, and that she wanted me to go on to work.

"You'll be taking plenty of leave later on," she reminded me. "You need to save it now! I'm perfectly capable of doing this alone, so please let me!"

Reluctantly I agreed and went to work while she went to the hospital. The procedure was to take approximately four hours.

When she returned to my house that afternoon, she looked good, but it was apparent that she was exhausted. She complained of feeling very cold, and it was difficult for her to get warm. She curled up on the sofa, I wrapped her up in a blanket with the heating pad, and before too long, she fell asleep.

As I watched her sleeping, I wondered what her dreams were like. Does she think about the cancer continually? Does she think about dying? Does her life play out like a movie? Does it seem real to her, or does she expect someday to wake up, and realize it was all just a horrible dream … a nightmare? I sometimes think that I'll wake up and realize we have all been in a time warp, and now things will be normal again. Maybe she does too. I prayed for God to give her peaceful sleep — dream-free — sweet and comforting sleep, refreshing her to face yet another strenuous day.

The next two days were very rough for Joy! She lost her appetite, and she would sleep for long periods of time when she returned from the hospital. She looked as tired as I had ever seen her. However, on the third day, she was given potassium and magnesium because it was determined that her electrolytes were wacky. What a difference that made! She called me after she left the hospital, and she sounded bubbly and full of energy! She even wanted to go shopping that afternoon to finish up our Christmas list. Once we arrived at the mall, she said she was really hungry, and she ate a real lunch, the most she had eaten for days. If one didn't know better, one would have thought she was perfectly healthy!

We began our shopping spree, did our usual "people watching," laughed and carried out our usual craziness, stopped at the candy factory, bounded from store to store and shopped for at least two hours straight!

She was drawn to a booth run by the Salvation Army which was sponsoring underprivileged children in our area. She chose the name of a child from their list of needy children. While I shopped for gifts for her, she shopped for the little girl whose name she had chosen. By the time she had finished, she had purchased two pairs of shoes (of course one pair of shoes had to be athletic shoes), a sweater, socks, underwear and, of course, toys! The pleasure she got from this unselfish act was evident by the look on her face as she excitedly showed me the gifts she had chosen, as well as the little angel Christmas tree ornament she had been given by the Salvation Army as a reminder of the little "angel" who had touched her heart. The following week as I hung the little angel on our tree, at her request, I knew that because of Joy's giving spirit and unselfishness, this little girl would perhaps have her first real Christmas. I thanked the Lord for my friend's compassionate and loving heart, and I prayed that the little "angel," who was unknown to us, would feel the love that went into the giving of those gifts, and would someday accept into her life the greatest of all gifts, Jesus Christ!

Chapter 25

A Little Bit Of Christmas

Finally, the long four days of the stem cell withdrawal were over, and we were going for a weekend to Longwood College for Adam's Christmas Concert. I was very thankful that Joy felt well enough to go. In fact, she felt very well with the exception of being very tired. She was so excited about getting to go on a trip. Even though it was to be of short duration, it would be a change of scenery, and away from the hospital; it would also be a little bit of Christmas for her. I thanked God that she was able to go with us! He knew that we all needed that time together — away from the harsh reminder of what was to come.

What a wonderful weekend it turned out to be! The dinner concert was beautiful and so uplifting. It was almost as if we were at a Christian college. The music was Christ-centered, and we felt the very presence of the Lord in the room. What a way to start the Christmas season! Mother was thrilled to be able to be there, and for Joy, of course, it was very special. We were all so proud of Adam, most especially his grandmother! Hearing him sing, and knowing what a testimony he was at the school, was such a great blessing to us. It's evident to all that Christ comes first in his life, and he truly lives His testimony every day. My eyes teared as I quietly sang along with the carols, and I praised the Savior for all He had done, and all He means in my life!

We went to church with Adam and his friends the next morning. Though Jim is a man of few words, I knew he was very proud of Adam as I heard the pastor telling him what a blessing Adam had been to their local church through his work with the youth. Jim, in turn, thanked the pastor for his obvious concern for our son. The Lord had clearly led Adam to the right church, and for that I was very grateful. We drove home that evening, happy and thankful, even though exhausted. We had already celebrated Christmas ... together!

The week of December 6 was to be a rest week for Joy before her long hospital stay. We finished our Christmas shopping that week, and we wrapped all our gifts, trying to keep things as normal as possible. She seemed to be feeling good and more like her old self again — laughing, acting silly (as only we can), and, as usual, ignoring her aches and pains as much as possible. She helped me finish the quilt I was making for Julie and Andrew, and we even managed to make a few cookies. Of course, talk of the transplant surfaced often during our times together. I tried to persuade her to believe that things would be normal again, and that we would get through the whole thing together. I tried and tried to reassure her; however, it was difficult to convince her of something that I, myself, was not at all sure of. I trust the Lord without a doubt, and I knew she was, and still is, in His hands. But I believe He realizes our inability at times to fully accept without question what we don't understand, to the point of not being, at the very least, somewhat apprehensive, even though we trust Him. I'm so glad He understands that part of our frailty. Sometimes we think if we ask God to take control over a situation, and we still feel afraid, that it's because we don't trust Him enough. But I was just as scared as she was, and I began to realize that she needed to know that. And so I confessed my fear to her, we prayed together for strength and peace, and I felt we were then ready to go into the next battle together with the Lord! I believe that my confession strengthened us both, and I thanked God for letting me see that!

Our Sunday service, December 12, was beautiful. Pastor Trefry led our congregation in a time of prayer for Joy, and a laying on of hands by our church elders. I sang her favorite Christmas carol, "O Holy Night," as she had requested. As we left the service, our church family embraced her, and assured her that their prayers for her would be constant. She was obviously moved by their compassion and genuine love. What a long way she had come from that bold and rebellious girl of fourteen!

That evening we attended the annual Christmas concert at Julie and Andrew's church. We were all blessed by yet another little bit of Christmas, and the marvelous realization once again of God's greatest gift to His children. Hearing the "Hallelujah Chorus," I was struck anew by God's majesty, and I felt it was just a glimpse of Heaven when "every knee shall bow and every tongue confess that Jesus Christ is Lord" (Romans 14:11). "Oh, Lord," I prayed, "perform a miracle in Joy's life. Let us enjoy other Christmas times together. Don't take her home just yet ... I'm not ready to let her go. Indeed, I'm not ready at all!"

Chapter 26

The Sting Of The Bee

A little bright canary yellow Ford Mustang with a black convertible top — that is what she had to have, and all she had talked about, ever since she had seen one in Luray at Thanksgiving. She just had to have it!

"It's me, don't you think?" she said with that famous sparkle in her bright blue eyes, the first time we saw it.

Jim and I took her to a local dealership a few days later to see one exactly like she had seen in Luray.

"What do you think I should do?" she asked Jim, as we hurriedly got back into our car and out of the extreme cold and wind. It was certainly not a good day to spend outdoors looking at cars, but she seemed oblivious to the weather. Her cheeks and nose were apple red from the effects of the cold, but her face was filled with enthusiasm as she waited for Jim's advice. I knew that he had hoped that she would wait on the car until after the first of the year when she would be out of the hospital and have had more time to look around, and then perhaps be able to get a better deal. I also knew that he perhaps realized she needed something to focus on right now — something that she could look forward to after she was out of the hospital. And so he told her how to go about getting the best possible deal, and if she had the money to buy it, then it should be her decision. Jim is very practical but I believe he wisely concluded that just maybe, "practical" was not the best in this case.

Joy took his advice as a "consent" and decided (because Jim, due to his work schedule, could not go with her) to ask her cousin, Bo, to help in making the best deal. With her hospital date only two days away, time was of the essence if she wanted the car before she was admitted.

Those next two days were very exciting for her as she anticipated the purchase of the car. The twinkle was back in her eyes as she talked about it, and I knew it was a good diversion for her. She hadn't even had time to think about the impending transplant. I thanked God for that, and also for the fact that He cares about every facet of our lives — even our material possessions are certainly blessings from Him — if we are His children.

Sure enough, two days later, the little yellow car that we named "The Bumblebee" became a reality. Joy burst into our house that evening, her face literally glowing, as she related to us her day at the dealership, and then she hurried off to have an early Christmas with her cousins. The next morning would come soon enough, and I was glad that her cousin, Teri, had chosen this particular evening to have all of the loved cousins celebrate Christmas with Joy. She would have little time to anticipate the next day!

Adam came home from college that same evening for his Christmas break. Again I thanked God for His timing! Adam would be home to help us with what I knew would be a very stressful time for us all. Jim had been working very long hours at the office and even longer hours at home in the evenings just to keep up with his tremendous workload. He was looking forward to having Adam work part-time for him at the office, as well as having him home to help me with Joy. We both thanked God for our son's willingness to help do anything we asked of him. He was always eager to be of service, and his smile, which can light up a room, was just what we needed!

Chapter 27

No Turning Back

The dreaded, but much anticipated day finally arrived — December 15, 1993!

"Six o'clock seems mighty early," Adam said, as he dragged himself up the stairs the next morning, still looking half asleep. Joy and I were fully awake, neither one of us having slept much. Jim was his usual jocular self, providing us with his wonderful dry sense of humor.

"Have a good time!" he joked, as he hugged her when we were leaving. "I'll be praying for you," he added, in his serious tone. She knew he meant it, as she quickly kissed his cheek and turned to go out the door, lest he see the tears in her eyes. "You'll be home before you know it," he shouted, as we backed out of the driveway. I had promised Joy that while she was in the hospital, I would wear the cross necklace given to her by her mother. As I slipped the chain around my neck, I prayed to God that she would indeed be home "before we knew it," and that He would give to each of us His all-sufficient grace!

As we drove off in the still darkness, I sensed the apprehension and fear that filled the car. As Adam drove, he and I tried to be cheerful as we made small talk and cracked jokes. Joy was silent for a time, lost in her own thoughts. Before long she could resist no more, and she joined in. The tension seemingly melted away, and soon we were all laughing and acting our usual crazy selves.

It proved to be quite a long wait after we arrived at the hospital and checked her in at the registration desk. I often wondered why a person has to be at the hospital two hours before a surgery, only to have to wait at least half of that time sitting around! However, we were still in such good spirits that the time passed by quickly. Soon the long wait was over, and her name was called. Before the nurse took her to the operating room, the three of us joined hands and prayed for wisdom for all who ministered to her and for His peace. She smiled at us as she was taken away.

"Lord," I prayed again, as I watched her go, "let her sense Your presence, and give to her once again that peace that is not understood by this world. Please do for her above and beyond all we ever hoped or dreamed."

Adam and I spent a very long day together, but I was glad for his company. Finally, late that afternoon, we were told the surgery was over and that once she was out of the recovery room, we could see her. We were then given her room number. Adam and I hurried up to her assigned floor to make sure that the nurses had granted our request not to have her put in the same room where her mother had died, for indeed the room number we had been given was on the same floor — the same wing. Thankfully, her room was not even on the same hallway! We thanked the staff, and we could tell by our conversation with them that they were caring and compassionate — just one more answer to prayer!

The doctor talked to us before Joy was out of the recovery room. He assured us that she had done very well during the procedure, and that she had to be given only two pints of blood. Considering that he had thought she might have needed as many as four or five pints, he seemed very pleased. I just thanked the Lord, again!

This part of the procedure had involved the harvesting of the bone marrow and the placement of yet another port to aid in the re-infusion of the blood stem cells, as well as the many other fluids that had to be given to her through her veins.

The doctor told me that the only problem he had encountered was that the port had to be placed in, of all places, her neck, in lieu of her chest! Of course, that would be much more uncomfortable for her at first, but once she got accustomed to it, he assured me that it would be no problem for her at all.

It was extremely hard to convince Joy of that when we first entered her room. Tears streamed down her face when she saw Adam and me!

"I wanted to wait until after the nurses left before I cried," she sobbed. "Look what they had to do!" she said, as she angrily pointed to her neck.

The anesthesia was still very much apparent; therefore, I persuaded her to close her eyes and try to sleep, and we would discuss it when she was more fully awake and feeling better. She grabbed my hand as if she were afraid that we might leave. I assured her that we would stay with her until she awakened, and as I held her hand, she closed her eyes and drifted off to sleep. I prayed and thanked God that she had gotten through this part of the experience which she had been dreading the most, and I asked Him to give her encouragement as well as strength for what was to be a very stressful next few hours, as it had just been explained to us by her nurse.

As the day wore on and the anesthesia began to wear off, Joy seemed much more accepting of the port in her neck. Actually, once she was fully awake, she was so glad the surgery was over that she began to laugh as we named it "The Claw." It was at that point that she realized she had a bladder catheter as well! I thought she would have an absolute fit, as the nurse explained to her that she would have to have it in place for several days!

"What?" she exclaimed loudly. "I can't leave it in that long!"

"Yes, you can!" I said, feeling a little exasperated and exhausted myself from the very, very long day. "You'll just have to! There are some things in this life that you have to do, and this is one of them! I don't even want to hear it! You have no choice, so just make the best of it." She didn't say she would, but she quieted down, and even she realized that she had no other alternative. She also realized that the sternness in my voice was only because I cared!

With that matter settled, we then discussed the fact that, as she had previously been told, she would have to sit for five hours on the two ten pound sandbags already in place under her hips and lower back. That was to help seal, with pressure, the two holes made by the needle used in extracting the bone marrow. The marrow had been removed and frozen, so that if the stem cell transplant didn't work, the bone marrow transplant could be tried. It was the doctor's opinion that for her the stem cell transplant was her best chance, but her bone marrow could be stored for up to ten years. I guess you could call it "insurance." She was grateful that the doctor had gone ahead and taken the bone marrow at the same time of the port implantation, so that only one surgery was required.

We got her to laugh when Adam and I gave her a stuffed cuddly reindeer who had his bottom filled with sand. Adam and I had purchased the little deer in the hospital gift shop while we were waiting for her surgery to be over, and we had named him "Ruffles," after a deer Joy had hand-fed during one of our picnics in Luray. She had named him Ruffles because she had fed him potato chips. We told her he was there to commiserate with her because he was also sitting on sandbags! She soon seemed resigned to the whole thing, realizing it was inevitable, and with that, she laid her head back on her pillow and drifted off into a somewhat peaceful sleep!

Adam and I unpacked all her belongings, organized her room and, when she awoke, got her to eat a little something so that when we were ready to leave that evening, she seemed to be in pretty good spirits. She was to begin her four-day continuous chemotherapy later on that evening. The next battle had begun!

"Oh, Lord," I prayed, "I am reminded of your faithfulness, and your promise never to leave us or forsake us. To that we now cling."

As we got into the car to go home, Adam placed a white bag on my lap. I opened it to find a little cuddly reindeer like the one we had gotten Joy!

"I knew you loved it, Mom," he said, with a laugh in his voice. (How could he have known? I had only played with Joy's little deer the whole time we had been waiting in the lobby!) "I bought it for you so you would have a deer to commiserate with you, too."

I couldn't speak for a while as the tears welled up inside, choking my words. I praised God for our wonderful son and for his compassionate, loving heart. The gift would do more than that for me, it would serve as a reminder of the time he and I had spent together that day in service to the Lord, while ministering to another one of His children. I fell into bed that night totally exhausted but thankful to God for so very many things. And with Jim's arms safely around me, I drifted into a blissful sleep.

Chapter 28

A Calm Before The Storm

The following four days of continuous chemotherapy proved to be much easier on Joy than either of us had anticipated. She did not get as sick as she thought she would. Of course, if you knew Joy as we did, this would not have surprised you at all. She would not even allow herself to think about getting sick. I truly believe that is the key to a lot of it — mind over matter! She just wouldn't even think about it at all!

Missing Christmas Sunday at our church was very hard for Joy. Adam's gospel quartet from Longwood gave a concert, and she had to miss it! However, Andrew videotaped it for her, and as usual recorded it to make it very personal to her, and when she viewed it she would think she had actually been there. He also has a great sense of humor, which she surely needed now. I thanked God for him and for Julie. They have been so very supportive of Joy, as well as to Jim and to me, especially now.

Monday and Tuesday were to be Joy's "rest days." We were able to pick her up from the hospital on a day-pass, so we decided to have our Christmas on Monday, December 20. I fixed the traditional turkey dinner (her favorite), the kids were there, Adam, Julie and Andrew, and we all had a great time. We had the tree, the gift opening, a fire in the fireplace, music — everything. As much as she wanted to feel normal, and as much as she tried for the sake of us all to be festive and cheerful, she couldn't hide the reality of how she really felt. At least, she couldn't hide it from me. I had seen too much and been a part of it too long not to know the signs. We had been friends too many years for me not to be able to see through the mask. I watched her smile and laugh at the kids in their attempts to make things good for her, for she had become a master in disguise at shielding them from the truth. She was in tremendous pain from a bladder infection she had gotten after her catheter had been removed, and that, along with everything else, would have made most of us extremely irritable. But by the grace of God, she held on to her sense of humor until after the kids had gone and the party was over!

As I helped her into a hot bath, something she dearly loved but couldn't do in the hospital, she began to cry while the mask slowly slipped away.

"I could get so discouraged right now," she sobbed. "But I just can't. Not now."

We both cried, knowing that this was only the calm before the storm, and feeling completely powerless. We knew that we must now, as never before, hold on to God's promise that we had learned to love so much not to let us "be tempted (suffer) beyond what you can bear" (1 Corinthians 10:13), and that He himself was suffering alongside us and interceding for us.

Later that evening, after we had taken her back to the hospital, I told Jim of her discouragement and tears (she would never have let anyone but me see her cry for fear that it would be a sign of her lack of faith). He reminded me that God did not promise all our days would be good, and that we must trust Him all the more on the days when they are not. I realized as we talked that Jim could also tell when she was discouraged and fearful. She only thought she could hide it from him, too. He said, "God is faithful, honey. Hold on to that."

Joy felt much better Tuesday. Jim and I went to the hospital and picked her up on another day-pass. She was ecstatic at the thought of being able to leave the hospital for even a little while. She joked with the nurses that she just might not come back. They told her how much they would miss her, so we laughed and promised that we would not deny them the pleasure of her company later that evening.

On the way home, the three of us joked around, having a great time, and for a while it was as if it were the old times when cancer was a disease that affected other people — not us!

After Jim had gone back to work, Joy and I spent the afternoon together resting, having girl-talk, and then fixing dinner together. It was a time reminiscent of better days. We tuned the radio to the "Oldies" station and "doo-wopped" and "lam-a-lam-a-ding-donged" to a favorite song, while acting crazy and dancing all over the kitchen. It proved to be most refreshing, after what we had been through the last couple of days. I thanked God for those hours of frivolity, because it helped lighten the heavy, heavy burden we felt.

All too soon the time had come to go back to face the beginning of the biggest battle yet! Shortly before she was to go back to the hospital, for what we knew might be a very long time, she looked at me and said, "If anything happens to me tomorrow, know that I love you and your family. You are the best friend I've ever had and...." She wanted to say more but she could not. The emotion was too great. I don't believe I could have endured hearing another word, because already I felt as though my heart would break.

"Everything is going to be fine. You will see," I replied, without looking at her. "God is not finished with you yet, girl." We hugged each other hard, and scurried to the car where Jim was waiting.

Once back at the hospital, Jim kissed her goodbye, had his usual upbeat words for her, and then waited in the car for me while I went to her room with her to help her get ready for bed. We talked for a while, and I knew she was very concerned about the stem cell re-infusion that would take place the next day. We prayed together, and then we cried together. She suddenly jumped off the bed and looked straight at me.

"Here we are," she stated emphatically, "acting like a couple of idiots, crying and carrying on. We've trusted God so far, and He's never failed. So what does He have to do to prove Himself to us? We must not doubt now!"

Again, she had managed to cheer me up, and show me truth that I seemed to have forgotten, ever so briefly. We agreed together to keep on trusting, and to quit our "crying and carrying on!"

"Thank you, Lord," I whispered softly on my way down in the elevator. "Give her strength, the doctors wisdom, and keep her close to you, and above all, let her keep that sense of humor! I commend her to you just now!" I drank in His word: "Trust in the Lord with all your heart and lean not on your own understanding; in all your ways acknowledge Him and He will make your paths straight" (Proverbs 3:5-6).

Chapter 29

The Re-Infusion — The Storm

The next morning Joy was awake early in preparation for the long awaited re-infusion of the precious new blood-stem cells into her body. It is a fragile, sometimes dangerous procedure, because the solution in which the cells are stored can sometimes be rejected by the body, causing serious complications. Therefore, the cells were to be very slowly reintroduced into the body intravenously and manually, by Linda (remember Morticia), the oncology nurse. The entire process takes approximately two hours. The patient is then monitored closely for three to four hours to make sure there is no rejection or complication.

I knew she needed me there, although I didn't tell her of my plans to do so. She had assured me the night before that she would be just fine! Adam and I arrived in her room just as the procedure had begun. When she saw us, I knew I had made the right decision, because she looked very tense! She immediately began to relax as I told her that at that very moment my mother was calling our church prayer chain, and everyone was beginning to pray for her even as we were talking. "God is faithful," I kept repeating over in my mind. I knew Joy was praying as I watched her eyes close. Not too long afterwards, a look of peace upon her face replaced the tension. I thanked God for the added strength He gives to her!

"Everything is just perfect," Linda kept saying as the procedure continued. "All your vital signs are looking just great." When it was over, the nurses marveled at how well it had gone.

"I know," Joy said confidently, with that ever-present smile visible. "Everyone is praying for me, even as we speak."

"Well, it sure did work," Linda replied. "Usually patients experience at the very least elevated blood pressure and heart rate, but you ... you are just perfect." We praised God so very, very much!

Joy had to be monitored for several hours by a nurse who would sit by her bedside. Since she looked so extremely tired, and I knew she would sleep, we left and went home for a few hours. The nurse who was to monitor her would be Stacey, a wonderful young nurse who had been so sweet to Joy since she had been in the hospital. She had immediately taken to Joy and would arrange, whenever possible, to assign herself to Joy. She told me that because of Joy's upbeat positive attitude, she was an absolute delight to be around, and she couldn't do enough for her! I felt as though I had left her with a sister. Stacey became very special to Joy in the following weeks, and I had cause to thank God for her many times!

The following day was a second re-infusion, and it went just as perfectly as the first one had! We praised our God for His grace.

The next several days went fairly well for Joy, except that she lost her appetite almost entirely, and she began having diarrhea. Everything she ate, including Jell-O, caused diarrhea. It was food in ... food out! I brought her food from home, although by the time I fixed what she had requested and got it to her, she had changed her mind, and she wasn't able to eat it at all! We tried everything — Jell-O, bananas, soup, and everything bland we could think of. The doctor ordered stool samples and tested them for infection, but none was found. However, for precautionary measures, IV antibiotics were prescribed. The antibiotics caused her to experience unbelievable nausea. Joy became very discouraged. I prayed for wisdom for what to say to her.

"It will get better," I would tell her. "We knew there would be days like this ... we knew it ... hang in there ... you just have to tough it out." Easy to say if you are not the one who is having the problem!

One day when the nausea was especially bad, she looked at me and asked, "Do you think people are still praying for me?"

"Of course, I do," I replied. "I know they are. I pray for you all the time."

"I know you do," she softly sighed. "But I mean other people. The people who were praying for me before. You know … we all say, at one time or another, that we will pray for people, but then sometimes we get so busy with our own lives that we forget. Do you think they have forgotten?"

I knew how true that was! I long ago realized how important it is to pray for someone when you have promised them you would. I try not to do that anymore, because I know people depend on those prayers. I have myself. I believe it is a very serious thing to promise that you will pray for someone, and then fail to do so. It is a broken promise to God, as well as to those who have mistakenly depended on you. This truth was now impressed upon me as never before.

"Of course they are," I assured her. "The phone at home rings all the time with people asking about you, and we keep telling them to pray. I know they are. Satan wants you to feel alone and abandoned, but that just isn't true! You aren't alone, and you certainly haven't been abandoned by God, or ME."

As usual she cheered up, even though the nausea and diarrhea were ever-present, and once again I could see a faint glimmer in her eyes!

Chapter 30

God's Christmas Timing

Christmas Eve and Christmas Day Joy had almost too much company for her own good. She was totally exhausted from the events of the previous days, and it was apparent that she really needed to rest; however, the company served to make the holidays go by faster and kept her from feeling so lonely. I knew it was especially hard for her because of the recent loss of her mother, but I also knew that perhaps this was God's way of making the holidays completely different than they had ever been before, thus easing the pain of this first Christmas without her. Again, I praised God for his perfect timing! It certainly would not have been her choice to spend Christmas in the hospital, and yet God sees beyond our choices or what we want, deep into what is best for us, causing us, when we reflect, to be so very thankful that He is in control.

It snowed Christmas night and created a lovely ending to a very beautiful day with our family. The snow made everything seem fresh and clean. It was a reminder that God's best gift was sent to make us fresh and clean before God, and all we need do is reach out and accept it. I thanked the precious Savior for getting Joy through a most difficult time, and for so many answers to prayer!

Chapter 31

Reality Check Once Again

The day after Christmas we watched by television as our Redskins lost another football game. Jim and I sat in Joy's room and watched the first quarter of the game with her before we had to leave to go to Julie's parents' home for dinner. The team started the first quarter doing so well, but things went from bad to worse. We joked that next year would be a new year for Joy and a new year for the Redskins — both back better than ever! From the look on her face as she waved goodbye to us, I'm not so sure she bought that, but she sure liked the sound of it!

The next day, December 27, she called the house early. "Bring the clippers when you come this morning," she said.

"The nail clippers?" I asked, having been awakened from a sound sleep, and not quite realizing what she meant. "No!" she stated, sounding annoyed at me. "I mean the hair clippers! You have to shave my head because you know I can't stand losing it this way! It is driving me crazy, and loose hair is all over my sheets and my clothes." She sounded very depressed, and I knew the time had come once again to deal with the very visible side effects of chemotherapy.

When I arrived at her room, she looked completely exhausted and emotionally drained. She motioned for the trash can as she lay on the side of her bed, and just as I brought it to her, she began vomiting. The antibiotics were once again making her sick. I called for Stacey, and she immediately gave Joy an injection to combat the nausea and vomiting. Before too long the medication began to work, and the nausea subsided, at least for a while. She then became very tired and sleepy.

After sleeping for a while, she woke up and wanted to get on with her haircut. She managed to sit up in a chair, although I knew by her unsteadiness that she needed more sleep. She closed her eyes and remained silent as I began to cut away her thick, curly hair. Tears streamed down my face, as great locks of hair fell to the floor. This was the third time I had done this, and it was no easier this time than it had been the first time. No! In fact I think it was even harder this time, because I never even imagined I would have to do this for her at all, much less three times in less than two years! It was such a vivid reminder of the awful disease we were fighting — the enemy that had tried for over two years to break our spirits, but had only served to bring us closer to the Lord, and more determined than ever to be more like Him. Yes, it had broken my heart, but not my spirit!

Once the job was done, she showered, while I changed the sheets on her bed and straightened up her room. Stacey helped me to clean up the hair that lay in large piles on the floor. She had such compassion for Joy and for me as well. As a nurse, I knew she had encountered this scene countless times, and yet she made me feel as though she were going through our pain too. I needed understanding at that very moment, and she ably supplied it. I thanked God for Stacey, again!

I had made a bandanna for Joy out of "Redskin" material, and as she lay in her freshly made bed after her hot shower, I placed it on her shiny head. She looked somewhat refreshed but very, very tired. Even then she smiled at the bandanna, and there were at least no visible tears this time over the lost hair, only a seemingly quiet acceptance of things that could not be changed.

Adam arrived to take me home, and I left knowing that she would sleep most of the afternoon due to her medication. As we drove home, the snow continuing to fall as it had all day, I thanked God again for Joy's unique spirit and His reminder to us through His Word that "even the very hairs of your head are numbered" (Matthew 10:30). He alone knew how many had fallen from her head that day. I know also that He cares, and "will neither slumber nor sleep" (Psalm 121:4).

Chapter 32

Recovery Begins — Slowly

Because of the snowstorm, the road conditions did not permit us to get to the hospital the next day, December 28. However, when I talked to her on the phone early that morning, her spirits seemed to be good.

"I wish you could come over today," she said, sounding a bit disappointed when I told her it was not possible. "I feel so much better, and I wouldn't be sleeping or throwing up today so we could really visit."

"I know that," I replied gently. "But I would rather be there when you need me the most, like you did yesterday. I feel much better when I can't be there, if I know that you are doing well, just resting, watching television, following the doctor's orders, and staying out of trouble," I said, while laughing.

She conceded that point, and agreed to try to spend the entire day resting. Joy was getting better. I could tell. She then told me Stacey had just posted her stats and her blood counts were up! She sounded elated as she read them off to me. Praise God! The news couldn't have been any better. As we finished talking, and I hung up, I knew that because of the good news, she would be able to really have peaceful rest that day. I felt very thankful!

I concentrated on the work that had piled up at home, but with a whole new attitude. I phoned the many people who had been praying for her, to relay the good news. Mom and I let them all know how much we appreciated their prayers and asked that they continue to pray. I could hardly wait to tell my sister, Carolyn, who had been away with her family for the holidays, about the encouraging stats. Being a nurse, she would be especially thrilled! She had been praying for Joy faithfully, as had her church, and I wanted to share with her. Indeed, many churches across the country were praying, and we had appreciated it so much. I had even been in contact with her best friend when she was in college, and she, as well as her church in Chicago, had been fervently praying for Joy. We needed all the prayer to continue, as we knew it would. God had been so gracious. It was a great day of thanksgiving to the Lord!

Chapter 33

A Lesson Learned The Hard Way

"You've got to get me out of here," Joy announced very defiantly as I entered her room the next morning. She was very fidgety and obviously upset. She tapped her fingers on the side of the chair and appeared to be on the verge of tears.

"Hey! You will be out of here before you know it with those great blood counts," I said, as I stood before her wall chart reading the new figures the nurse had posted that morning.

"I'm going crazy! This room is driving me up the wall, and I know I would be much better if I could just go home," she stated in a loud voice, practically screaming!

I suggested this would be a good time to take a walk, and she agreed. She put her mask on, and we began our walk. Luckily, we ran into her oncology nurse, Linda.

"Well, don't you look good!" she said, with a big smile on her face.

Joy promptly spoke up. "Yes I do, and I think I am ready to go home. Now!"

"Well, well!" Linda said. "That is a good sign that you are certainly getting better. But it would be entirely too risky to send you home just now. Your counts do look good, but not good enough to release you from here yet. You surely don't want to go home only to have to come back, do you?"

Joy looked disappointed, but she knew in her heart that Linda was right, and it was confirmed by the doctor later on that morning. Maybe, he told her, she could go home next week. I reminded her that we could not complain about a few more days, when she had been so blessed. It was a gentle reminder, without preaching her a sermon, but she needed to hear it. She agreed, and after the doctor told her she could leave the floor to go to the cafeteria for lunch, providing of course that she wear her mask, we embarked upon what would prove to be a very long first trip for her!

She was delighted to be able to at least leave the ninth floor, so I secured a wheelchair, and we were off. It was apparent, even before the elevator reached the first floor, that this had not been a good idea. She was extremely weak. She had been telling me that the physical therapy the nurses were asking her to do was next to impossible for her. Yet even knowing that, I don't think she was fully aware of the extent of her weakness! I know I certainly wasn't. It didn't take either one of us very long to get the "big picture."

In the cafeteria, I took her to a table, and then went to get the BLT and French fries that she wanted. Once back at the table, I couldn't believe my eyes! She looked absolutely terrified! She did not speak a word as she attempted to eat her sandwich, and she avoided any eye contact with me or any of our surroundings. She broke out into a sweat and was visibly shaking.

"I have to go back now," she said sounding like a frightened child, her eyes filled with fear!

"Okay," I replied, gathering up our half-eaten food and trays. "I'll be right back for you after I throw this away."

As we went back up to the room, neither one of us spoke. I knew she was on the brink of tears, and I knew she did not want to cry in public. So I just got her upstairs as quickly as possible. It was so hard to see someone who had, not very long ago, been so independent, now so weak that she had to be pushed in a wheelchair, and too overcome with that realization that she couldn't even eat! It was one of the saddest moments I had ever faced with her.

Back upstairs, she fell into bed, and I prepared to leave so she could sleep. As bad as the experience had been for her, it had made her painfully aware that she was not ready to go home yet. She had to wait a while longer. She needed to see that for herself, and I thanked God that He allowed her to come to that conclusion and to be content with it. It had been a hard, but necessary lesson for her to learn! Waiting always is!

Chapter 34

Another New Year

Friday was New Year's Eve, and our annual church New Year's Eve party, always held at our home, was to go on as usual. My heart wasn't in it this year, because Joy would not be there. She was always a big part of it.

Jim and I worked hard all day to prepare the food, and get everything ready. Our usual fare was chili with all the fixin's, sandwiches of several kinds, salads, chips, sherbet, and homemade desserts. We usually made several kinds of chili. We had "not hot," "hot," and "hot-hot"! Joy always made the "hot-hot" chili (she claimed it was "not that hot!"), and everyone always looked forward to trying her chili. I tried to add a few more drops of hot sauce to one batch of chili that I made, just so the tradition would not be broken, but it wasn't the same — nothing was the same!

With both Jim and me working together, cooking, chopping, baking, and so on, we were finished in record time. Joy had called several times to see how we were doing, all the time wishing she could be there. By late morning, she had developed a fever, and the doctor put her back on IV antibiotics. She began to sound discouraged. I knew the fact that she couldn't be a part of the celebration didn't help the situation at all. It was hard to encourage her when I felt so discouraged, but I did my best. Later in the evening just before our guests were to arrive, she told me she was extremely tired and really felt like she could sleep. And indeed she did sleep — almost the entire evening. Stacey, bless her heart, cut the ringer off on her phone, and she had uninterrupted sleep for many hours. She needed the sleep for so many reasons. One, the nausea was so bad that she needed sleep to help her cope with that. Secondly, the sleep helped her not to think about what she was missing at our house. I thanked God again for His blessed gift of sleep.

The church crowd was smaller than usual, which added to the disappointment of the day. However, during the devotional part of our evening, I couldn't help but be filled with praise to the Lord as we had special prayer for Joy. And as I looked around the room, I counted so many other blessings: my friend, Mary Rose, who is now in remission from leukemia; my own dear mother who was in recovery from congestive heart failure; my son, Adam, so sick last year, and so healthy this year; his girlfriend, Rita (visiting with us for a few days), a wonderful Christian girl with whom we had all fallen in love; my son, Andrew, and my daughter-in-law, Julie, building their lives together, and making Christ the head of their home; and most importantly, Jim, so supportive, so rock-solid, such a source of strength. As 1993 drew to a close, I could do no less than "praise God from Whom all blessings flow." This year had been most difficult, and yet we had all grown from the difficulties. What would this new year, 1994, bring? I prayed for strength for what was ahead for all of us. "May we be lights in a darkened world, Oh, Lord, may we live each day with no regrets, and may our lives count for You."

Chapter 35

Let's Just Praise The Lord

The next day was Sunday, January 1, 1994. Just as I arrived at church, there was a message for me to call Joy at the hospital.

"Guess what?" the excited voice on the other end of the phone said, when I returned the call. "My blood count is up to 600, and the doctor said I can probably come home Wednesday! Tell everyone at church that I want to hear their praises to God all the way over here."

We indeed did praise God that day for His continued care for Joy and for our many, many wonderfully answered prayers!

Over the next two days, January 2 and 3, Joy encountered high fevers, followed by antibiotics, nausea, more antibiotics, platelets, and so forth. Amazingly, her spirits were up because, despite everything, she was confident that she was going home, and she was sure it would be very soon. That was all she talked about. I tried to get her to realize that it may not be as soon as she thought, so she wouldn't get her hopes up too much, only to have them dashed, but she wouldn't hear of it.

"I'm leaving Wednesday ... I promise you," she would state emphatically!

Tuesday evening Joy's temperature was 101.4 and she was again on antibiotics. When I called her, she seemed to be somewhat depressed but not hopeless.

"I'm waiting for the doctor to come in now to tell me if I can go home tomorrow. I just have to go home ... I just have to!" she said, sounding more irritated than anything else. Actually, more spirited, and more like her old independent self.

I said, "Be reasonable. You don't want to come home only to have to go back, do you?"

"I'm not ever coming back!" she said unequivocally. She hung up rather irritated, but I laughed and praised God for her high spirits. Not long afterwards, she phoned and sounded much more subdued and reasonable, even though she had received the official word that she could not come home yet. She had accepted this small setback, and I promised to visit her after work the next day.

I prayed all day that her temperature would remain normal, and that perhaps she could still come home; however, the day came and went, and it became obvious she would not. We were disappointed, but not dismayed. She assured me that it would be THURSDAY ... "NO DOUBT ABOUT IT!" It was refreshing to see her old fighting self re-emerge. It was a sign — a very good sign!

Chapter 36

Uncle Hairy

Uncle Hairy was now ready for the competition! Who is Uncle Hairy? He's a ceramic head that, when spread with seeds, is supposed to sprout "hair" in a few weeks! Joy and I had purchased him before she went in the hospital. I decided we would have a contest to see who grew their hair back first — Joy or Uncle Hairy. Now that Joy's hair was officially gone, it was time to prepare Uncle Hairy. Today, January 5, 1994, the contest began!

I called Joy when I got to work, to try to cheer her up by telling her that Uncle Hairy was ready, when she smugly informed me that she could come see for herself because she was given the word from the doctor that she could come home! I gladly told her I would make arrangements to come and get her as soon as possible!

As excited as she was, she was also apprehensive, in part because of what had happened the day we went to the cafeteria at the hospital. We talked about the incident, and the fact that it had occurred because her blood counts were still very low at that time, causing her tremendous weakness. Now she would find that, because her counts were up significantly, she had more strength, and now the doctor felt she was prepared to leave the hospital!

"Uncle Hairy" seemed to lighten the mood, as well as our talk about the arrangements to get her home.

As we left the hospital later that day, and with the old twinkle in her eye, she turned to me and said, "Did you know that if you ice a bald head long enough, you can lower your body temperature?"

I looked at her in complete astonishment; however, knowing it was utterly useless to scold her, we broke out into fits of laughter, as she recounted to me her unbelievable antics, and I pictured her bathing her head in crushed ice all night, so the nurses could not record a fever! I just prayed to the Lord that He would take care of her, and He did, for she never developed a fever after that day!

I thanked God for her determination and her ability to see beyond herself to what God desires of her, and I prayed for her and what would lie ahead in the following days, months and even years, for it appeared this battle was now over at least for a while!

Chapter 37

The Road Back To Normal

Joy recovered remarkably from her stem cell transplant. We were so hopeful that this would be her "cure." She admitted to me that it was the most difficult thing she had ever been through, and despite all her attempts to cover up her pain and agony during those last long weeks, I had known that to be true. I had seen through her stoicism! I prayed for this to have worked in her body!

She quickly began to regain her strength once she was home. Her hair soon began to grow back (curly once again). She remained at our home until we felt she was able to cope on her own. I knew that until she got back to her own place she wouldn't feel "normal." For Joy, "normal" is a misnomer! She has the inordinate ability to make herself feel "normal" as long as her surroundings are familiar — friends, church, home, work, and so on. She will not allow herself any "lag time," as she calls it. She has too much living to do, and she intends to make every minute count.

Oh, that we all could do that! If we could but grasp that truth — that we have only the very breath that is in our nostrils at this very minute, and that we could be facing eternity with the very next one. How differently we might live! So many times that breath is used to complain, lie, gossip, curse, fight, boast — the list is endless. And we, as Christians, are as guilty as anybody! Unfortunately, and all too often, we do not use that precious breath to encourage, soothe, heal, love, praise. There are days that we don't even use one moment for praise! We are all guilty. I am guilty!

"Oh, Lord, may we see our failures and never cease to praise you. May we use the breath you so graciously give us to honor and glorify You. Thank you for allowing Joy to experience that truth, and for teaching me, through her example! It is a gift that I cherish!"

Chapter 38

Back To Work — A Calm Settles In

Our family, including Joy, of course, enjoyed another of our fabulous beach vacations — her love! We even got Jim to take a ride on the waverunner — not a long ride, but nevertheless, a ride! We had a great time, and shared great laughs! Joy was in surprisingly good health. We were very hopeful that the stem cell transplant had been successful!

Our church softball season, 1994, came and went, and Joy coached another winning team!

She insisted that she could play. She would bat, and if she was successful in making it to first base (and unfortunately for me she usually did), I was to be her designated runner. Yes! The bottom of the barrel had been scraped, and I was pressed into service. Needless to say, my over-fifty-year-old bones felt every jolt as I ran the bases trying to score. You see, I am not at all athletically inclined, but for the good of the team (at least two women had to play at all times according to league rules), I have subjected myself to all forms of ridicule by my appearance on the softball field. Actually the team is very kindly toward an old lady and has encouraged me in this endeavor! We have had some great times, as I have graciously allowed the team to enjoy many laughs at my expense.

It was so good to see her playing again even if it was in a limited capacity. I praised Jesus!

It was also during this hot summer that we moved Joy into a brand new condominium! It was the first time she had owned her own home. Jim had been urging her for some time to consider owning her own home instead of renting. She finally bit the bullet, so to speak, and she selected a condominium not far from her apartment.

Jim and the boys and I helped her move in (the air-conditioning broke on moving day!). I stenciled most of the rooms for her, and she and I stored up many more "Lucy and Ethel" memories as we worked together for hours at a time, laughing all the while at our unorthodox methods of using ladders, paint, nails, and so on.

With all of our family working together, we had her "at home" in a very short time!! It was a blessing to see her still living one day at a time while trusting the Lord to be there. You see, we really do not have to worry about tomorrow because God is already there! She continues to be a living reminder to us of that truth!

Of course, Joy was back at work as soon as the doctor had given her the clearance, but earlier than he would have preferred! However, one soon tires of her constant nagging and whining (ha, ha) and, therefore, out of desperation, he relented and she had gone back in early spring. Normal! Remember what I said? She had to feel normal!

Work! Well, that is a story in and of itself! Joy has worked at NBC studios in Washington, D.C., for approximately eighteen years. I have touched on this very briefly before. However, since she has had cancer, her whole purpose for working has changed.

She loves her job and there is no doubt of that. Her major in college was education. She planned to teach physical education in high school, and she would have made a terrific teacher. But God had other plans for her. She landed a job at NBC through a friend. She never really intended to stay there. She wanted to teach! The months and years went by and she become "hooked" by television.

In this regard, Andrew and Joy are kindred spirits. Andrew has his degree in Mass Communications. He loves the field of radio and television, but it is very competitive. He went through a period of struggle when he found himself without a job at one point. He and Julie drew much closer to the Lord and to each other during that dark period in their lives before the Lord provided by giving him a very good job in his chosen field. We grew closer together as a family as we went through that time with them. But as Julie and Andrew were faithful to Him, He answered prayer above anything they ever hoped for! Our jobs are important to God. He places us where we can best serve Him. We need Christians in all walks of life, whether it be in the Christian or secular world. What better place for a Christian than in the media!

Joy has worked her way up at NBC, and now works at the Network Research Library. She has been assigned exclusively to President Clinton. Her duties include thoroughly screening videotape of the President's daily activities and updating information in the NBC Archives Computer. She researches videotape of specific people, places and events for use in such shows as *Nightly News, Today Show*, and *Dateline*. Her other duties consist of providing footage of particular events, people, and so forth, as may be necessary for producers who are doing news stories. It is a very exciting, but often stressful, job. She has continued to work all through her battle with cancer and has only used leave when absolutely necessary for surgery, her stem cell transplant, and her now weekly chemotherapy sessions (she only misses the actual day of chemotherapy).

Her work continues to make her feel "normal." She is still as reliable as she has always been at NBC. As a rule, she shows up early each morning and stays late whenever needed. She was recently named "Employee of the Month," an honor that she is very proud of.

Her life has been an inspiration to many people at the station. Many of her co-workers who are experiencing family or friends who have cancer have sought her advice and have questioned how she has maintained her spirit! She has been able to witness effectively because she has not let cancer RULE her life. It is truly just a diversion from her real purpose in life.

In January, 1993, Joy was invited by the news staff at NBC to go to the White House with them while they did a story on the President. Joy was thrilled, as was her mother, for that opportunity. I have always been glad that her mother was alive when that happened in Joy's life. Her mother was especially proud of Joy and God allowed her to be able to share in that special moment in her daughter's life. I gave her a hard time because of my Republican convictions, and we shared a good many laughs over it, but the "President" is the "President," and I display the picture of her and the President in my office!

What an exciting job! What opportunities she has had to witness! Praise God!

Chapter 39

A Small Setback

The end of September, 1994, Joy began to experience pain and swelling in her left shoulder. We feared that it was the return of the cancer!

A trip to see the doctor, however, revealed a blood clot in her shoulder. It was caused by an infection that had formed in her implanted port.

The port was surgically removed immediately! She was placed on blood thinners, and I had to give her shots of heparin to help dissolve the clot. She was so relieved that it wasn't a return of the cancer that she didn't even think twice about the surgery!

We praised God for everything, including the weekly blood test results which were great. A bone scan was to be scheduled after the clot had been taken care of. We continued to feel God's presence!

The fall came and went, and we celebrated another Thanksgiving together. Joy continued to live each day to its fullest, as she just accepted God's will for her — one day at a time! All who know her were, and still are, amazed.

Chapter 40

"Lucy And Ethel"

It was at this time, fall of 1994, that Joy decided it was time for us to launch into a new adventure. We had found these lovely cloth and gold bead necklaces at a craft fair we had attended and she was convinced that if I took one of them apart to see how it was assembled, that we could make them, sell them for Christmas presents, and make some Christmas money!

I have always maintained that I couldn't sell umbrellas in the rain, but seeing her enthusiasm and remembering the Christmas of 1993, I agreed!

If you knew of only some of our past ventures, you would have laughed even before we began! We have wallpapered until 2:30 in the morning, shingled a roof (under Jim's supervision), painted, landscaped, changed our first flat tire (unfortunately, without Jim's supervision), sorted eggs at a chicken hatchery (reminiscent of the Lucy and Ethel candy factory episode), and, our greatest feat, pushed a 300-pound carton containing an unassembled computer table up a flight of stairs in order to hide it from Jim, as it was to be his Christmas present! That venture alone was worth a television sitcom episode, for we had seen our counterparts do similar things countless times!

First of all, the day we chose to purchase the computer table was bitter cold! We arrived to pick the merchandise up at the store in Joy's Mustang convertible. The man who met us at the loading dock just looked at us in disgust. We were not dissuaded though. We simply took the top down and asked him to load it into the back seat, as though we had carefully thought it out, which, of course, we had not! Once it was loaded in and we drove off, we put on our sunglasses and pretended we were going to the beach!

"This way we won't feel so cold," Joy quipped.

No! It didn't help, but the giggles and the stares we received all the way home sure did!

Once home, we had to decide just how to "lift" this thing out of her car. I stood on the back seat and together we flipped it, as carefully as you can "flip" a 300-pound box, out of the car!

"Okay," I said. "Now what?"

We managed, with the help of a hand truck, to get it from the car to the house and even inside the front door! When we looked at the long flight of stairs leading up to the second floor, we both sat down and laughed!

"Can't we just leave it down here and let the guys take it upstairs after Christmas?" Joy said, knowing full well what my answer would be.

"I can't do that!" I tersely replied. "It's a surprise. Where would you propose I 'hide' it down here?"

"I know. I know!" she shot back. "It was just a wild thought!" she continued, with a smirk on her face. She then slowly but convincingly said, "We will push it up the stairs one step at a time using our backs and our backsides, of course, and pushing it with our feet," she stated, sounding very confident.

"Okay," I agreed. "We can do it!"

It was much easier said than done! Imagine us sitting on the steps trying to push 300 pounds up the stairs and realizing that if it slipped it would push us back down the stairs and smash us into our beautiful grandfather clock which so far was still standing in the foyer below.

Of course, my just mentioning that brought tears, caused by our uncontrollable laughter, to our eyes! We then became ridiculously silly and we laughed so hard as we moved it inch by inch, that several times we lost ground by slipping down a step or two instead of moving up.

We eventually got to the top step where she abruptly pushed the full weight of my body onto the top of the box, forcing it to lay flat on the top step. We had made it!

We both lay there laughing as we caught our breath. One would have thought we had climbed Mt. Everest if one had heard us gloating over our ingenuity! We then pushed the box down the hallway, into the spare room and under the bed, where it stayed until Christmas morning when we proudly retold the story of the eventful day to the family!

Lucy and Ethel, as we are often known, had once again been successful and prevailed.

Therefore, given a bit of our background, we felt that indeed we could now enter a new venture — SALES!

Little did I know just how successful we would be! I was a bit fearful as I walked into my school and took the first ten necklaces with me.

"You don't want to buy any of these necklaces, I suppose?" I stupidly said to my co-workers as I entered the main office on the way to my clinic. Great salesperson that I am!

I didn't even get through the office when, to my surprise, all ten were sold and I had taken orders for at least five more! The venture became a nightmare. Everywhere I went in the building, someone had heard about the necklaces or had seen one and wanted to buy one or more. One lady even bought nine at one time! I got calls, visits, referrals — teachers and staff members that I didn't even know called to place orders. They were all buying Christmas presents!

Every evening I would go home, Joy would come over, and after dinner we would go upstairs to our "Santa's Workshop" and cut, sew and bead necklaces. It became a joke. We couldn't make them fast enough (remember Lucy and Ethel and the "Aunt Martha's Homemade Salad Dressing" episode?). When someone suggested that we make earrings to match, I almost cried. We got so tired of the "Workshop" that we dreaded another order! When it was all said and done, we had made over 100 necklaces! When we could stand it no longer, we closed Santa's Workshop for 1994. No! We do not plan to open up next Christmas!

Our little venture did yield some pretty nifty Christmas money, and for that we felt pretty smug. However, I still to this day can't bring myself to wear one of the little numbers!

I have thanked the Lord many times for these memories. Most people do not experience memories such as these in a lifetime. We have crammed a lot of memories into what might be remembered as a very short time. My family and I often sit around and recall all of the silly times we have shared with Joy and with one another. Those memories are some of God's richest blessings to us!

Chapter 41

A Crushing Blow

As Christmas, 1994, approached, Joy began experiencing swelling in her left knee. An x-ray revealed that the cancer had surfaced once again — this time in her femur!

Even though I knew that she had suspected it for some time, when the doctor called her with the diagnosis, it was a time of dark discouragement for her as well as for me!

We had, of course, been praying for a healing for her — maybe at least a remission! All of our devotions of late had reminded us that God's timing is not ours, but I still felt very discouraged and very much afraid for her.

Her doctor's appointment was set for December 8 and I had planned to go with her to find out the course of radiation treatment to be followed.

I spoke to her on the telephone the day before her appointment and I felt her fear and disappointment as she cried to me over the phone.

"I'm so sorry that I am crying," she softly sobbed. "I guess I'm just losing it and I can't let that happen!"

I tried to offer comfort but I didn't know how. "We must remember, above all, that God is still in control and we must trust Him. You keep telling me that and I know you believe it, so now is the time to appropriate the strength He gives and has given all along." I spoke those words hoping against hope that my own discouragement was not apparent. "There is nothing wrong with tears. God expects them and He understands. It's okay. We will get through this together." As I hung up the phone, I, too, cried as

I felt her pain. I was reminded of a poem written by James Whitcomb Riley titled "The Old Fashioned Bible." He wrote it while reflecting upon the death of his dear father:

... The blessed old volume! The face bent above it —
As now I recall it — is gravely severe,
Though the reverent eye that droops downward to love it
Makes grander the text through the lens of a tear ...

Sometimes our tears can act as a lens through which we can see more clearly that which we could not see before. I had seen it happen over and over again in the past few years, and I knew it to be true. The tears were necessary and they, too, were a blessing from our Heavenly Father!

I called Joy later on that morning and she was bubbly and bright. I thanked God again for the cleansing tears and the peace they bring forth!

My own fears were yet another story. I wanted very much to understand, but I had a very hard time doing so. I felt at a total loss. I questioned why she wasn't in a remission — just a remission. We have many non-Christian friends who are watching our lives and I didn't want to belie my testimony. I can't let them know that I feel angry ... discouraged ... disappointed!

I prayed for wisdom. I needed to know how to cope. I knew God was in control and that He was faithful. How could I help her? I needed wisdom then more than ever before. I couldn't let her know how discouraged I was!

My devotion for that next day centered on faith — faith that God will do as He has promised. But I also remembered He promised "... that if we ask anything according to His will, He hears us. And if we know that He hears us — whatever we ask — we know that we have what we ask of Him" (1 John 5:14, 15), and I didn't feel secure in that promise! Later on I realized that I had failed to put enough emphasis on the "according to His will" part of that verse! It was simply that at that point nothing made sense to me at all. How could I minister to her with my terrible mindset? "Oh, Lord," I prayed, "I sure do need direction!"

Sitting with Joy that afternoon in the doctor's office was a grim reminder of what might be ahead for her. I remembered all too vividly our first trip there, and how I felt as I looked around the room and saw the other patients in their various stages of this disease! I wondered how each of them was coping with their situations ... how many of them had the Hope that I knew Joy had.

It was then that God showed me the way that I would cope! Joy leaned over and whispered to me: "The pastor told me that when Jim gave everyone my latest report at prayer meeting Wednesday night, a cloud seemed to come over the congregation. See, that's just what I don't want to happen! I don't want people to always see the bad and awful side of cancer. I want them to see that good comes out of it, too. My life has changed for the better through my cancer. I am a different person because of it! God has answered so many prayers for me. This is His will and I have accepted it. I want people to see Christ through my cancer!"

That was my answer! She had managed to encourage me and to give me strength. I knew then how to help her. We discussed how her witness through her cancer had already been manifested to her co-workers and at my school to my co-workers, also. Not to mention the testimony she had been at church and with our neighbors as well. She said if her cancer had caused her to be able to witness more effectively, then so be it! I determined to help her in that witness. I could not ... I would not cheapen it by a poor testimony to those who were watching our lives. We were responsible to that "great cloud of witnesses" who were watching us "run the race" (Hebrews 12:1).

Chapter 42

A Return To Square One

As Joy finished her radiation, it was time for another bone scan. (By this time we were very familiar with the routine!) Her knee was much improved, at least pain-wise, and she was feeling pretty good. What a disappointment when we got the results of the bone scan! The cancer had metastasized and had invaded both shoulders, both knees, her spine, her breastbone — the stem cell transplant had not accomplished what we had hoped! She was to begin a new chemotherapy, Taxol, immediately.

Taxol is a relatively new type of chemotherapy. It paralyzes the support structure inside the cancerous cell, rendering it unable to perform any functions necessary for growth or reproduction; therefore, it dies.

Because her port had been removed earlier, due to the blood clot, Joy was told she would have to have another port surgically implanted before the Taxol therapy could commence. She would not have to be hospitalized to get the chemotherapy (Intracare, here we come again), and the series would not begin until after Christmas! Joy rejoiced so much with this news that even her doctor seemed amazed at her attitude! He had seen it before, but this certainly seemed completely unbelievable, even to him!

The cancer had not been stopped. She would have to have even more aggressive chemotherapy. She would lose her hair again, would still suffer untold side effects, but she would not be denied another Christmas! How I marveled at her complete trust, her assurance, and her complete yielding to His will! What lessons I was learning from my young friend! What a gift she had given to me! Joy talked with me about this latest turn of events with a calmness that only comes from the Lord and complete reliance upon Him. She related to me her devotions of late about blooming where you are planted — no matter where that may be!

"I know that my temper and my impatience have sometimes hurt my testimony at work," she confided to me. "I want to change that. I want to take every opportunity God gives me to witness for Him. I know that I haven't always done that. I have gone to work when I have been so tired and when I didn't think I could make it, but that has been my choice, and it doesn't give me the right to snap at people and lose my temper and shame the Lord, as I sometimes do! As long as God gives me life on this earth, I want to use all the opportunities He gives me!"

I felt guilty and ashamed because I knew that I had missed many opportunities also, and that my time on this earth could be even shorter than hers might be, because none of us knows when God will call us home! I also became committed that day to strive harder to make the use of every opportunity. We were both growing, even though we hated the vehicle through which He had chosen to accomplish it!

And Christmas? It was blessed.

Chapter 43

"Courage"

Joy had her new port implanted surgically on January 9, 1995. Her first treatment of Taxol began January 18. The treatments continued through the months of February and March and the first two weeks of April.

She, of course, lost all of her hair again. This time when she requested a hair cut, I gave her a "mohawk"! We laughed as we went upstairs to show Jim, the boys and Julie. How many times had I cut her hair? I had lost count! But God, in His wisdom, had taken her beyond even that, and she willingly accepted it.

During this time, Joy's cough started up again and it became uncontrollable! A further trip to the doctor and another chest x-ray revealed fluid in her lung. Up until that time, she had been taking antibiotics and cough suppressants to no avail, because the doctor confirmed that the fluid was not an infection, but was cancer related!

Joy was also informed at that time that the Taxol she had been taking was obviously not working. She took that news with a calmness that now had become "normal" for her.

"Well, what's next? Am I going to die soon?" she matter-of-factly asked her doctor!

"No!" he sharply replied. "We have some other things we are going to try," he said, sounding frustrated rather than annoyed by her question. "I had certainly hoped that the Taxol would have worked, but there are other things. We are going to put you back on 5FU therapy, but unlike the 5FU you have had before, it has a vitamin added. The purpose of the vitamin is to break up the cancer cells into smaller ones that can be more easily attacked by the chemotherapy. I would like to start you on it this week, that is, if that fits into your schedule," he joked. "And, you can receive the treatments right here in my office … no hospital … no Intracare!" He added that, knowing that those words alone were like music to her ears!

I could sense the frustration and disappointment in his voice and see it on his face, as he talked with her. He, as well as all of the nurses and staff in his office, had grown to love Joy. They marveled at her spirit. They had all been hoping for a cure for her. With each new treatment that she was given, I knew the thought was always the same — maybe this one will work!

The first treatment of the "new and improved 5FU" was set for April 21. Blood tests revealed that her red blood count was very low, and therefore I had to commence giving her injections again — three times a week until her chemotherapy was completed!

We left the office together, but this time there were no tears and no quiet talk on the way home … just an acceptance of what was to be. Strangely enough, I felt a peace inside my heart, too, although I can't explain it.

The injections were very painful — much more painful than the ones I had given to her previously. Because of that, it became increasingly more difficult for me. She would cry and then declare she was taking no more of them. Then we would both laugh and she was all right until the next time! She decided on her own after several weeks that she would take no more. Enough was enough! It hasn't seemed to have hurt her at all. What a relief for her as well as for me.

Her hair began to grow back after the Taxol was out of her system. One day she decided she needed to have that little bit of fluff on top of her head colored, for it had turned grey! I told her I could do that! No problem! And so that evening Miss Clairol and I gave her a dye job!

"Oh, no!" I said to myself when I had dried it. The color wasn't exactly right … it was a beautiful … light … ORANGE!

The kids were there, and we couldn't keep from laughing. All of a sudden she cupped her hand, brushed it across her nose, and said, "Courage! I need a little courage!" She sounded just like the lion in *The Wizard of Oz*! Of course, the kids went into fits of laughter and that word has since become a family joke! She even recorded a message on her answering machine at her home which ends with "Have a little ... courage!"

I thanked God for the memories we continued to make, even though they were laced with sadness. I know we will remember them fondly in the years to come!

Chapter 44

His Eye Is On The Sparrow

Spring 1995 and Joy's chemotherapy continued. She continued to take her treatments once a week. The x-rays, the scans and the blood tests continued! She continued to work, we continued to go on as normally as possible and everything continued and continued and continued! She continued to praise and thank the Lord and I still continued to feel helpless. I cannot fix it. I'm much better at yielding, and I don't question like I use to, for I am learning. But I sure would like to "fix" it!

My mother had been having health problems of a different nature for several months — something about which I knew nothing — DEPRESSION! I have since learned that depression is very common among the elderly. It is something else that I could not fix, even though I tried very hard to do just that!

After going through a series of doctors and tests, we were led to Christian counseling where she received marvelous help — help from those not only medically trained, but grounded in Christian principles as well. She is on the road to recovery!

Our family is still going through a very difficult time. Depression can devastate a family just as surely as cancer — it affects every member. But with prayer and help, I know that we will emerge victorious. Some day I must tell you how God worked in my life through this experience. My faith had been tested once again but God is faithful!

Just when I felt that I could handle no more, our son, Andrew, lost his job. My heart cried out to God, "Where are you?" Joy was no better, my mother was in a constant state of depression, and now this.

I cannot tell you that I prayed and that things got better right away. In fact, for a time, things just got worse. I didn't see how that was possible, but it happened!

Then one day my devotions centered on the story of Abraham and Isaac. God seemed to speak to my heart and ask me what I was withholding. Abraham had not withheld even his only son (Hebrews 11:17): "By faith Abraham, when God tested him, offered Isaac as a sacrifice." What was I withholding? I realized that I was holding on to my will ... my independence. I needed to give that to Him and become totally dependent upon Him. I could not continue to try to fix things by myself. He knew that I was burdened, and carrying a heavy load, but He also knew that I could handle it if I allowed Him to guide and lead.

I would love to tell you that I immediately did that, but the flesh is weak, and it took a while, but when I was finally able to yield, God took over the situation, and the burden was lifted! I praise Him for his sustaining power!

That summer, I was taught a valuable lesson by the Lord, a lesson that I could have learned in no other way. He used His creation to teach me what He had been trying to teach me for some time ... that He doesn't need me to fix anything! He is sufficient!

A pair of wrens chose our front porch to build a nest and raise their family. Now, I just couldn't understand why they chose a place so open, so noisy, and so vulnerable. The mother and father wrens worked feverishly building the igloo-type, tight-knit little nest. It was an amazing piece of architecture, to say the least! Our family, including the dog, continued to go in and out the front entrance as usual, even though I tried to encourage them to be very quiet when they opened or shut the door. We continued to gather on the front porch swing and glider, as is our custom during the spring and summer months. We laugh, giggle, and talk, sometimes being joined by a neighbor or two. It can get very noisy, and yet our birds did not seem to mind in the least, once they realized that we could be trusted. They flew in and out of the nest at will.

Soon after the little nest was completed, the mother wren laid in it seven lovely cinnamon-colored speckled eggs! I couldn't even imagine how two birds could fit inside that nest, let alone seven!

One morning I noticed that one of the eggs had been placed outside of the nest. I toyed with the idea of placing it back inside the nest, but I have always heard that if you touch the eggs, the mother will not return to the nest. So I left well enough alone. After all, I reasoned, with one less egg, there would be a little more room for the other birds once they were hatched.

We kept a close watch on the eggs for several days. Joy, Julie, Mom and I were quite excited about the prospect of baby birds. The guys seemed a little less enthusiastic, although they reported many times to us the whereabouts of the mother, after we expressed alarm when we hadn't seen her for a time.

Then one very hot, 100 degree day, we looked in the nest and saw several fluffy little birds! They were so small that we couldn't tell how many of them there were! They just looked so hot! They were all crammed into that small little nest! How could they survive the heat? I became very concerned, and even placed a small container of water on the arm of the porch swing, hoping that the mother wren would use it to give her babies water. I even thought of misting the nest ... it was so hot! I worried all that day about those babies. I looked in the nest frequently to check to see if they were still alive. The mother wren never took up my offer of water. I was beside myself! I concluded that they couldn't survive ... not in the extreme heat, for the next day was just as oppressively hot.

You know what? Those six baby birds grew, flourished, and flew out of that nest, all without my help! God didn't need my help with those birds, and He certainly doesn't need me to fix anything for Him! All He wants me to do is to be willing to be used when He calls on me ... willing to be ready to obey Him. He also doesn't need me to tell Him how to fix things, although I have on occasion. And He doesn't need my advice!

That beautiful old song, "His Eye Is On The Sparrow," has never meant more to me than it did then! If He cares about the birds — my little wrens — then how much more must He care about Joy — about all my family — about me!

Chapter 45

The Victory Is Pure Joy

And so it goes, more tests, more treatments, more x-rays, more scans, different treatments, and yet, this has become Joy's way of life. She just incorporates these "minor inconveniences" into her everyday life ... now, without question!

And yet, her testimony grows stronger with each passing day regardless of her condition. She never asks the doctor about her prognosis. I don't believe she really cares anymore. Oh, she would love to be in remission, or better yet, cured! But her eyes continue to be focused on her real purpose in life ... that of glorifying Jesus Christ, no matter what the circumstances! She is, without a doubt, living as the apostle Paul did when he wrote in Philippians 4:11: "For I have learned to be content whatever the circumstances."

It remains to be seen who the victor will be or who will win the war, at least in the eyes of the world. However, we already know who the victor is! Joy has won, and she is victorious through Jesus Christ, no matter what happens to her earthly temple! Her life and testimony have changed the world by changing the lives of others. Many have seen Jesus through her, because this whole ordeal has indeed made her to be more like Him!

She has changed my life, and that of my family as well. We thank God for the privilege He gives us to be able to minister to her, for she has enriched all of our lives. We, as a family, have grown and matured in the Lord, along with her. We have found strength in our love for Him and for each other. We will truly cherish each new day that He allows us to enjoy with Joy, and we will never cease to praise Him. We are confident that "as for God, His way is perfect ..." (2 Samuel 22:31).

More Like Him

You were just a girl when we first met
Was it so long ago?
You had a smile — that winsome smile
That set your face aglow.

You were most rebellious I do recall —
Mischievous and bold,
But deep inside, beneath it all,
I knew your heart was gold.

I couldn't help but hear the call
Of God to be your friend;
To do my best, with love and prayer
To win your soul for Him.

And so with gentle guidance
And God's compelling love,
You gave your life to Jesus
And He wrote your name above.

Much time was shared together
Reflecting time and time again
On the truths I taught within God's word,
To make you more like Him.

You abided my teachings and chiding as well —
We grew from teacher and student to friends.
I think you knew I only wanted
The best from you, for Him.

Now you face a challenge in your life
Far greater than them all,
And the world's amazed at the strength you show
as upon His strength you fall.

You've grown in Him beyond belief
From the young girl I first knew.
You're living proof of God's sufficient grace
He provides for me and you.

You've become a blessing to others —
The Lord Jesus they can see.
Now you've become the teacher
And you are teaching me ... that

Whatever God has planned for us
We know for sure, my friend,
That it will be whatever it takes
To make us more like Him.

S. Rice
1993